MW00522698

*Weaving practical instruction
and first-hand knowledge together
with Doug's personal experiences makes*
The Diabetes Antidote *more engaging than
the typical fitness guide or medical advice book.
Doug's own success establishes the credibility
of the approach he recommends.*

The Diabetes Antidote's *greatest value
may well be in what it offers those millions
of people who haven't yet developed Type 2
diabetes but are headed in that direction.
Doug's "exercise prescription" truly
can be an antidote to the development
of this lifestyle-induced condition.*

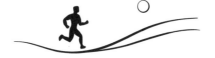

THE
DIABETES
ANTIDOTE

An Exercise Prescription
To Prevent Type 2
To Combat Type 1

by Doug Burns, Mr. Universe

with Denny Dressman

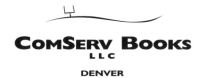

COMSERV BOOKS
LLC
DENVER

Copyright © 2007
Doug Burns and Denny Dressman

All rights reserved.
No part of this book may be reproduced in any form
or by any means without permission in writing from the authors,
except for brief quotations embodied in critical articles and reviews.

For information, contact
ComServ Books
P.O. Box 3116
Greenwood Village, CO 80155-3116
www.thediabetesantidote.com

The Diabetes Antidote
LCCN: 2007925076
ISBN-10: 0-9774283-1-1
ISBN-13: 978-0-9774283-1-1

Production Management by
Paros Press
1551 Larimer Street, Suite 1301   Denver, CO 80202
303-893-3332   www.parospress.com

Book Design by Scott Johnson

Printed in the United States of America
1   3   5   7   9   10   8   6   4   2

The Diabetes Antidote

To my little girl, Emily,
the sweetest-hearted girl I've ever known,
with an overload of talent and shine;
To my Aaron,
strength personified, a true comedian, and
owner of one of the best voices I ever heard;
To my Jordan,
total maverick, unrelenting trouble, and
intelligent beyond your years.

D.B.

For Brent,
who also dislikes "empty playgrounds,"
and hikes, bikes, skis, skates,
swims, fishes and tosses ball
with Erika and Rachel
every chance he gets.

D.D.

Foreword

By *Andrea L. Hayes, M.D.*

Hayes Endocrine and Diabetes Center

Nashville, Tennessee

OUR SOCIETY IS experiencing a devastating epidemic. Almost 70 percent of our population is now considered overweight or obese, contributing to the 8 percent of Americans who now have diabetes. It is estimated that 12,000,000 Americans are diagnosed with diabetes; another 6,000,000 remain undiagnosed. Unlike potentially lethal infectious disease epidemics in our country's history, there is no known pharmaceutical cure for this disease of our times. Nor will there be one in our foreseeable future.

Although the prognosis, at first thought, bodes bleak, in fact the most effective medical treatment lies within the power of each individual. This treatment does not cost hundreds of dollars monthly; actually, it is free and available to everyone. What is this magic secret? You will find out in this book.

As an endocrinologist, I and my health care team treat thousands of patients with chronic medical problems related to unhealthy lifestyles, a poor diet, and lack of appropriate physical activity. We write hundreds of prescriptions aimed at improving such common conditions as diabetes, high cholesterol, high blood pressure and others that may eventually lead to the leading killer in our country – heart disease. Insurance companies reluctantly pay for some of these expensive medicines; our insurers rarely fund preventive therapies.

While that's the bad news, the good news is stated within the pages of *The Diabetes Antidote*. We all have the ability to make lifestyle choices, including what types and quantities of energy we consume and the energy that we expend through activity every day. What you will find in this book is a straightforward approach to health improvement delivered with passion and practicality.

I have seen many patients become the victims of their own circumstances in living with diabetes, which unfortunately leads to devastating complications if this disease remains uncontrolled. Doug and Denny's approach is to educate, motivate and inspire their readers.

Occasionally I meet someone who asks me the question, "Do you suffer with diabetes?" They really mean, "Do you 'have' diabetes?" as if everyone who carries this diagnosis suffers. My resounding answer is always an emphatic "NO!" Living with diabetes does not guarantee suffering any more than buying a treadmill guarantees fitness. Take a look at Doug Burns, Mr. Universe, and you will not see a picture of a man who suffers!

The field of diabetes has exploded over the last few years and offers us more tools than ever to treat this epidemic. We have new and improved blood glucose meters, insulin pumps, blood glucose sensors, and designer insulins, as well as a plethora of pills targeted at insulin resistance, insulin deficiency, and the body's disposal of glucose once it is ingested. We sometimes find ourselves giving patients hundreds of units of insulin per day, only to find out that some individuals can "out-eat" even the most sophisticated of insulin regimes! Alternatively, caloric restriction can dramatically reduce insulin needs by improving insulin resistance in a matter of only a few days! We now have oral agents specifically designed to reduce insulin resistance. One side effect, however, is WEIGHT GAIN, of all things! So, as a health care provider, I find myself frustrated in achieving the results that I strive so vigorously to achieve.

It is my hope that *The Diabetes Antidote* gives you the tools, the knowledge and the motivation that are required to achieve a sense of empowerment for your health. You will be inspired by the obstacles that Doug overcame, starting at a young age with the diagnosis of diabetes. You will see that anything is possible if one keeps the vision and the faith. Set your goals and keep focused on the inspiration that you read through these pages. The rewards and pride that you will achieve will be greater than you could ever imagine.

In good health,
Andrea L. Hayes, M.D.

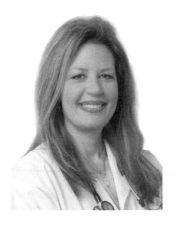

DR. ANDREA L. HAYES developed Type 1 diabetes at the age of 15. Her personal experiences with this disorder led her to specialize in this field of medicine. Her private practice, "Hayes Endocrine and Diabetes Center" in Nashville, Tennessee, has provided excellent care for large numbers of patients for the last nine years. She is actively involved in clinical research and serves as a national speaker educating health care providers regarding the treatment of diabetes and obesity. Her weight management program, "The Nashville Solution," has helped patients lose as much as 150 pounds. She is actively involved in The American Association of Clinical Endocrinologists and the American Diabetes Association.

Her favorite hobby, of course, is EXERCISE!!

Introduction

MAYER B. DAVIDSON is a respected and accomplished physician in his specialty, endocrinology. His long and distinguished career, which began with a degree from Harvard Medical School, has established him as one of the nation's authorities on the management of Type 1 diabetes and the prevention of Type 2.

Dr. Davidson has served on the editorial boards of leading medical publications, and has written hundreds of articles, book chapters, reviews and abstracts. He has been a contributing member of the American Association of Diabetes Educators and The Endocrine Society, and has received prestigious awards for distinguished service in his field.

At this point in his career Dr. Davidson serves as director for the Clinical Center of Research Excellence at Charles R. Drew University in Los Angeles, and is a professor of medicine at the UCLA School of Medicine.

Dr. Davidson was president-elect of the American Diabetes Association when I met him in the late 1990s, shortly after I had won the title of Mr. California in the California

State Physique Championships. I had been invited to speak at the City of Hope National Medical Center's first national diabetes conference in Duarte, California. Dr. Davidson was on the program, as well.

Prior to this conference I met with Dr. Davidson in his office. He was a kind and generous man, showing me around and introducing me to his colleagues. We began conversing about the importance that exercise plays in the lives of those faced with diabetes. I was surprised to find this renowned physician stymied by one aspect of his practice.

Dr. Davidson explained to me that many of his patients were under the impression that if exercise was so vital to both controlling and preventing their diabetes, then surely he, their physician, would write a prescription for exercise for them.

"Doug," he told me, "I'm not an expert in exercise. Medicine is what I know. Medicine is what I practice."

And then he summarized the problem he was facing.

"As the doctor, I'm believing the patients are taking care of their own fitness needs," he explained. "But the patients are believing that the doctor should be taking care of their fitness needs. There's a huge gap in between these misconceptions."

As a Type 1 diabetic since early childhood, and as someone who has learned firsthand the critical role exercise plays in limiting the devastating effects of diabetes as well as preventing the onset of Type 2, I could appreciate the doctor's consternation.

But I wasn't expecting what he said next.

"Doug, you need to step in and fill that gap," he told me. "Be the voice for us in the medical field, and be the voice to those with the disease, about the major importance that exercise plays in their lives.

"You need to deliver the message: Exercise and the fitness lifestyle are a life-saver for those with diabetes. For those predisposed, they make up the unspoken liberator."

ABOUT 550 PEOPLE attended the City of Hope National Medical Center's first national diabetes conference. Near the beginning of my presentation, I asked the group for a show of hands to see how many in the audience had diabetes. It appeared about 90 percent of the people there raised their hands.

For the first time, I asked how many knew the difference between Type 2 and Type 1. Hands, of course, went up again.

But when I called on some of those in the audience and asked them to explain the difference, they couldn't do it. They'd say something like, "Oh, yeah, uh . . . Well, one you get when you're older, right? And one you get when you're younger."

I used that little audience participation exercise to try to get across the point that Dr. Davidson had made with me. It was my first attempt at giving an exercise prescription.

The physicians on the platform nodded their agreement as I stated, "It's not your physician's responsibility to take care of you." I told them, "If you have good health, you can certainly thank your physician. But if you have bad health, you certainly can't blame him or her. The onus is on us." By the end, I think most of them understood this too-often-unspoken rule, that *we* are responsible for our own health.

I've made many appearances since then. Always, be it to elementary school children, medical conferences or stadium presentations, the exercise prescription is the focus of my message. The reaction I consistently get is the reason I decided, finally, to write this book.

"Where can I get a copy of your book?" I have been asked repeatedly. People are always surprised when I answer, "I haven't written one." The message to me was clear: "Then you should."

When I finally decided to attempt a book, I thought I'd call it "The Exercise Prescription" for several reasons. It was short and catchy. It implies help, intervention, or treatment. And it sounds authoritative and credible; experts "prescribe."

But after considering the powerful impact exercise can have in the lives of everyone who is managing Type 1 diabetes, and the undeniable capability of exercise to prevent the onset of Type 2 and in many cases even reverse it, my co-author, Denny Dressman, and I switched to "The Diabetes Antidote," and kept the "exercise prescription" as part of the subtitle.

A widely accepted definition of *antidote* is *anything that relieves or counteracts an injurious effect.* That certainly describes the role exercise can play in preventing Type 2 and treating Type 1!

THIS IS NOT the autobiography of Mr. Universe 2006-2007. But I will tell you about myself as we go, because my experiences as a record-holding strength athlete, world champion bodybuilder and prominent personal fitness trainer, and my experiences as a Type 1 diabetic since the age of seven are the basis for my conviction that exercise *is* The Diabetes Antidote. I hope my story helps you to become a believer, as well.

I've committed to making this as succinct as possible. My message isn't really that complicated. It doesn't require a thick volume of examples and instructions, with illustrations and how-to photos.

It's also important to understand that, although I have won both the Mr. USA and Mr. Universe physique competitions and have set American records in weightlifting, you don't have to aspire to any level of competitive achievement to benefit from this book.

If you are among the tens of millions of Americans who are at risk of developing Type 2 diabetes and want to avoid that fate, or if you are among those living with Type 1 or Type 2 and want to reduce the risks we face while enjoying a fulfilling life, *The Diabetes Antidote* can help you accomplish your goal.

If you feel like the circumstances in your life are making it impossible for you to change, please let me show you how to make those circumstances work for you. Whether you were just diagnosed, have had diabetes for a few years, or like me, have had it for decades and over most of your life, you can actually use the situation to better your life, reduce the medications you use, and in many cases get off of them altogether.

I'm not throwing theories out to you. I have put together the components of fitness that I know to be effective, the same ones that have won me championships. They work for me and for the clients who have chosen me as their trainer to help them succeed.

With that, let's get started.

1

Exercise as therapy

> ' . . . for those of us with diabetes,
> sustained regular exercise
> can actually reduce the amount
> of insulin our bodies need
> to function efficiently.'

I WAS A skinny, scrawny seven-year-old – other kids referred to me as "the bag of bones" – when my Type 1 diabetes was diagnosed in 1970. And diabetes management was an inexact science, to say the least.

Blood glucose monitors had not yet been developed. Insulin pumps didn't exist, either. And doctors generally thought exercise was a bad idea for anyone with diabetes. I actually had a doctor tell me I should not exercise!

Back then, your blood sugar level was determined by testing your urine. It wasn't a very effective method. Partly because of that and partly because my body was starving for food, I'd eat everything I could, including breaking into the nurse's fridge at school and stealing the little ice cream cups. I had very poor control of my diabetes for several years. I was in ketoacidosis on a regular basis because of my consistently elevated blood sugars.

In case you're not familiar with the condition, ketoacidosis occurs when the body starts breaking down its own fat for energy instead of using the glucose in the body for fuel. This happens when your body lacks the insulin it requires to transport the glucose from your bloodstream and deliver it to your cells. Your liver keeps pumping out more glucose, but your body isn't using it. Ketoacidosis is a serious condition. It can be fatal.

By the time I was ten, I had been taken to the hospital by ambulance some 30 times, and another 20 or so by my parents. This is a very abnormal amount, even by the standards back then. Most of the time it was due to ketoacidosis, but occasionally it was the other extreme, insulin shock. I was in the hospital so much, I failed fifth grade, which added greatly to my low self-esteem at that time. I had been labeled an "extremely brittle diabetic," meaning my glucose levels would fluctuate erratically. Due to elevated blood sugar levels and the inability to get the needed sugars inside my cells, my body was literally feeding on itself. My body was simply wasting away, and it showed.

The school I attended required all students to wear uniforms, and that was a problem in my case. My mother was not able to find shirts small enough to fit me. My pants were usually buckled up around my sternum, with my belt always locked on the last hole. I looked like someone or something from a Jim Carrey movie or a "Saturday Night Live" skit. My arms were so thin I could touch my thumb and middle finger around the middle of either one. I had become so small and skinny that doctors recommended injecting me with Growth Hormone to help me grow. It was decided against, but I wished like crazy that they had done it.

At the age of ten years old, I was brought to the emergency room at Johns Hopkins Hospital in Baltimore, in probably my worst condition ever. I had a blood sugar of 1153. That's almost ten times the high end of the normal range, and easily could have been fatal. It was the second-highest blood glucose they had ever seen at Johns Hopkins to that point in their history, and still might be.

As I was placed on the examining table and the nurses removed my clothes, my waist was so sunken that I couldn't see it while lying flat on my back. The emergency room physician asked the nurse my vital signs. These were questions I was accustomed to hearing, but on this particular occasion I remember the nurse looking down at me with sorrow in her eyes and holding up a folder to hide her voice so I wouldn't hear her. But I heard her anyway.

"He's only 56 pounds," she whispered. When I heard the sadness evident in her voice, I didn't know what to do. But I knew this was not a "normal life." I wanted out. I hated the way I was out of control, and the way I looked. I had been bombarded with all the general statistics about diabetes. Your chances of heart disease, stroke, and circulatory impairments (and the eye and foot problems that result from poor circulation) are drastically amplified, sometimes by 300 to 500 percent. But fear is not the best way to get anyone to make lasting changes.

Shortly after my stay at Johns Hopkins, I was back in DC Children's Hospital in Washington. I had exhausted physician after physician, and they told me if my elevated blood glucose levels continued, I would go blind, lose my kidneys, and die at a very young age.

They brought me down to the kidney center, where you could see some of the people who looked as if life had already left them. I still remember the place and the feeling I had inside. The doctor led me to a man with scraggly hair who had had one of his legs amputated. He was connected to a hemodialysis unit used to filter his blood.

I knew what was coming. I knew the doctor was going to tell me that if I continued to let my sugars remain high, I

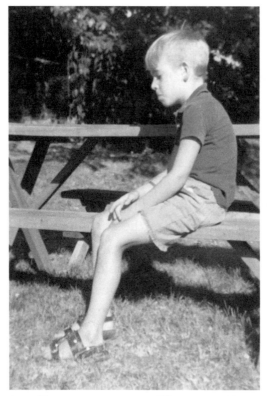

DOUG AS A SCRAWNY 10-YEAR-OLD.

would become just like that poor man. My initial thought to myself was, "Yeah, right. He's *old.*" The doctor obviously read the expression on my face. He simply said, "Suit yourself," and walked away. That doctor never knew, and probably never realized the impact that "tough love" had on me. But he gave me just what I needed. I did not understand the risks I was creating for myself by being so out of control, but I knew I was messing up, and I knew that only I could change things for the better. Soon after, I made the decision that changed my life and probably saved it, too.

I had seen that familiar advertisement of the day on the back of a magazine, the one that showed the guy down on the beach with the pretty girl, touting that you didn't want to be "a 98-pound weakling." Except for me as an 11-year-old kid, I was sure my world would be better if I could only *increase* my weight to 98 pounds! I figured at that weight I'd be able to fend off all the taunting and abuse I received at school and become a semi-normal kid.

I decided on my own that I was going to lift weights and get as strong as I could. But my parents told me I first had to get my doctor's approval. When my mom and I visited him for a regular check-up, she announced: "Douglas wants to lift weights, but I don't think he should." The doctor agreed.

After an uncomfortable silence, I got up the nerve and asked him, "Why not?" He answered: "It isn't healthy for someone with such a severe case of diabetes." I didn't think he had really answered my question, so I again asked, "But, *why* not?" And he responded, "Because it isn't healthy."

I was angry. It appeared that he either thought I was too dumb to be given a legitimate answer, or he didn't have one. I stuck out the emaciated sticks I had for arms and said, "It's healthier to look like this?" It was a survival response. I no longer cared about anything other than fixing my sickly self, and I knew I was going to lift weights with or without his support. I didn't know then just how important exercise is to a person with Type 1 diabetes, or why. But I do now.

TYPE 1 DIABETES puts a strain on many parts of the body, both internal and external. Exercise helps strengthen every one of the affected areas that Type 1 diabetes either has burdened, or has attempted to burden. With the fitness lifestyle, you can alleviate the onset of peripheral neuropathy (reduced sensitivity in your feet and hands). You'll keep your kidneys in check. Your heart becomes much stronger. Your venous system, your arterial system – all of those things – benefit greatly from exercise. There's no doubt about it.

That's the whole reason the initial advice I had from that physician when I was a child was such an influence in my life. Intuitively, it didn't make sense. I said to myself, "Well, you know, exercise is a way to get healthy, and I'm the epitome of unhealthiness." It just didn't make sense.

He was advising me not to exercise, because it was a risk; because I was so unhealthy, he thought exercise would destroy me. I understood him to say, "You can't do it. You have a disease, and it's going to work against your health," when the truth is, exercise is exactly what I needed, physically and emotionally.

It's the same principle as the therapy you'd go through to recover from an injury. It used to be that when athletes had an injury – pro football players, sprinters, soccer players – the advice was to rest only. The team physician would have you rest. It was the same advice following most surgeries, including some really major ones. Even new mothers were kept in the hospital for days and spent most of their time in bed.

That's no longer the case. About 15 years ago, a physician said, "You know, I bet moderate exercise would help an injured player recover." Since then it's been an ever-advancing practice. The benefits that aerobic activity provides, both as a tool for healing and as a preventive measure, are recognized and accepted everywhere. It increases the circulation, so the damaged area is being fed the nutrients it needs to recover much more quickly. The toxins that are in the system are being released at a much quicker rate than if you're just sitting still. Most importantly, you become part of the solution instead of becoming a passive victim. Every part of your body and mind is vital in working out your recovery.

Now for those of us with diabetes, sustained regular exercise can actually reduce the amount of insulin our bodies need to function efficiently. That might surprise you. It might even cause you to doubt me. But think about how the cells of your body get their fuel.

You've eaten that piece of bread or some rice or that banana – whatever. It's gone through the digestive tract and has been converted to glucose, and it's in the bloodstream waiting to go somewhere. The cell's receptors are waiting to receive it. The insulin is transporting that glucose out of the bloodstream and moving it into the cells.

That's one way. But there's another way. *Exercise.* It's the other method of getting glucose into the cell. When muscles are being used, they're requesting glucose at a higher than normal level. In effect, the muscle is saying, "I need it. I need it." It's using it right away, and the higher the level of activity, the more glucose your body's going to use and need. This is great news! After the workout, you've taxed the muscles, and now they're very depleted. The glycogen has been spent during the workout, and the muscles need to recover.

Exercise has facilitated consumption of the glucose. It's acting like insulin. It's just that it's somewhat unannounced. The view used to be that the effect of exercise was minimal;

insulin is the only glucose mover. It *is* the *primary* mover, but you can get the body to respond with exercise, too. When that exercise reaches a certain point, suddenly your body has become a metabolic machine, and to varying degrees, this is what we're after.

This doesn't mean you have to be engaged in extreme activity. You don't have to be training to be Mr. Universe or set powerlifting records. Anyone who wants to achieve their weight loss or fitness goals must continue to advance the stress they put on themselves. It can be gradual, but continuous nonetheless. This isn't an opinion. It's a basic physiological process. A muscle placed under new stress adapts by improving its ability to handle the stress.

Here's how it works. Each muscle is composed of tiny muscle cells, and during the workout the muscle cells have stress placed on them and undergo micro-tears. The more work, the more weight and the shorter the rest times all require more muscle fibers to become recruited, and more breaking down occurs. Immediately after you stop the stress, your body takes the protein it has available and converts it into specific amino acids, reconfigures them, and applies them to the damaged muscle cells. The great part about this is that your body over-compensates, and builds the cells back a little stronger. This is why athletes keep moving up their workout levels.

If you keep doing the same thing, day in and day out, the muscle will never change. It doesn't need to. It's acclimated to the stress that you're giving it. So to advance, whether your goal is to lose 25 pounds, or you're preparing to compete in an athletic event, or you're simply trying to improve your basic level of fitness, you have to keep advancing the resistance placed on the muscle. When you do this, it keeps regenerating, coming back a little stronger. This is how you become stronger and fit.

It doesn't matter who or what your competition is: yourself, another person, an obstacle you're trying to overcome, or a goal you're trying to achieve. If the stress a person imposes on himself or herself doesn't change or advance, there is no reason for the body or the mind to change or advance, either. It's similar to reading the same chapter in a book, over and over. You may enjoy the material, but to advance intellectually, you must read another chapter, another book, and move beyond what you've already learned.

The key for someone with diabetes is stepping over the mental barrier to get out there, to get started. Then it becomes getting your body to recover better. And that means keeping your blood glucose levels under control, because when your sugars are high, the process is going to be interfered with. Cell walls become rigid, and that impedes blood flow through the small vessels around the muscle or other tissue that is trying to recover. If the flow of red blood cells is impeded, the release of oxygen and nutrients is impeded, which lessens the recovery.

As I share my experiences and my views about exercise and its importance in combating diabetes, I often think back to that time when I marched defiantly out of my doctor's office to begin lifting weights. Several years later, after I had set an American record in the bench press and had received some local news coverage, I saw my former doctor in a grocery store. He came up to me, congratulated me, and laughingly said, "I see you didn't follow my advice about avoiding exercise with your diabetes . . . and I'm glad you didn't!"

We chatted for a few minutes, and he apologized. But, he said, at the time what he told me was the standard and accepted protocol.

How things have changed for the better as far as medicine's views of exercise and diabetes are concerned! I only wish society's habits hadn't gone in the other direction at the same time.

Antidote Reminder

Exercise greatly benefits your physicality and emotional strength. Check your sugars before you begin exercising, during your exercise, and after, too.

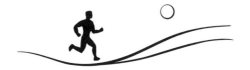

2

Thwarting Type 2

'. . . with Type 2 diabetes,
genetics may load the gun,
but inactivity and being overweight
pulls the trigger.'

WHEN MY DIAGNOSIS of Type 1 diabetes was made, there was not one diagnosed case of Type 2 diabetes in a child, anywhere. Not one. Thirty years later, a panel of experts convened by the American Diabetes Association estimated that 20 percent of all of the children newly diagnosed with diabetes were diagnosed with Type 2. Twenty percent. Some estimates are as high as 45 percent.

Here are some more numbers that help define the shocking scope of the problem. According to the most current statistic available, 18.2 million Americans have diabetes. That's more than six percent of our population. Of those 18.2 million, no more than ten percent – fewer than two million – have Type 1. That leaves almost 16,000,000 with Type 2. And, the Centers for Disease Control project, one of every three Americans born at the start of the new Millennium will develop diabetes in their lifetimes. For most, it will be Type 2.

The audience at my City of Hope presentation, the one that didn't know the difference between Type 1 and Type 2, was by no means an exception. I am continually surprised to find that so many of the people attending the conferences where I speak still think Type 1 and Type 2 are pretty much the same thing. So let's start there.

Diabetes Mellitus is a metabolic disorder in which the body's ability to produce or utilize the hormone insulin is impaired. But there is a big difference between the two types, and those of us with Type 1 are very aware of the difference. While many people with Type 2 had been walking around for months, sometimes years, before being diagnosed, the onset of Type 1 is drastic and severe, and must be treated immediately. Both types revolve around use of insulin, which is produced by the islet cells within the organ called the pancreas. Sugars from various foods that we eat are converted into the simple sugar glucose and absorbed in the bloodstream. Insulin is responsible for transporting the sugar from the bloodstream into the cells of the brain, muscle, and fat through cell receptors.

Type 1 diabetes, a.k.a. Insulin Dependent Diabetes and Juvenile Onset Diabetes (juvenile diabetes for short), is considered an autoimmune disease. The body secretes antibodies normally used to combat viruses, but in those of us with Type 1 diabetes, the body's immune system mistakenly targets and kills the insulin-producing islet cells of the pancreas. This leaves us with little or no insulin being produced. A person in this condition has now become insulin dependent, and injections of the hormone are needed to stay alive.

Type 2 diabetes, a.k.a. Non-Insulin Dependent Diabetes (formerly Adult Onset Diabetes), is a different ball game. With Type 2 diabetes the body still produces insulin, but the cell receptors that enable the insulin to function have become sluggish or non-responsive. It results from a genetic predisposition to its development, along with several other factors, most significantly the lack of exercise, being overweight and poor eating habits. Most often, Type 2 is treated with oral medications, though some Type 2 patients do end up on insulin injections.

For decades Type 2 showed up almost always in middle to later adulthood. But our Twenty-First Century lifestyle is changing that. It's no secret that as our activity levels declined and our consumption of carb-laden artificial foods including hydrogenated "trans-fat" poisons escalated, our incidence of Type 2 diabetes skyrocketed. Is that coincidental? We know it's not. "You see the effects throughout the world; in places like India it's become a pandemic," a physician friend from Diabetes India points out. "Inactivity has become commonplace; carbohydrate-laden diets are the norm; and the occurrence of Type 2 diabetes is at levels never before heard of."

ONCE I FINALLY achieved better control of my diabetes, growing up was a lot of fun for me. We had moved to Mississippi by then. Virtually every day of the week, after homework was done, my friends and I either hiked and explored the local swamps or organized pickup football games in two park fields nearby. Every single day something was happening. The playgrounds were always full.

I was recalling my childhood activities during a flight to Florida for an ADA conference in Orlando after I'd won the Mr. U.S.A. championship. I was looking forward to seeing playgrounds filled the same way I remembered them from my childhood. Shortly after I arrived, I passed by a couple of parks. Both were completely empty! It made me think about a park I pass regularly in California, and I realized it never seemed to have kids playing in it either. For me it was the realization of an alarming trend.

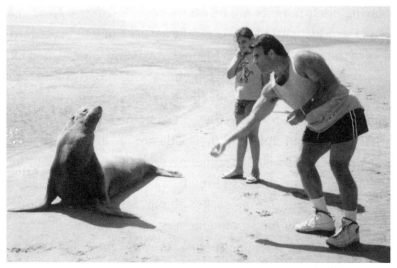

DOUG AND DAUGHTER EMILY AT PLAY ON THE BEACH.

When I returned home, a friend of mine named Tracey, who was a student at the University of San Francisco, told me about her idea for a term paper she had to write. The title, she said, was "Empty Playgrounds." Tracey was thinking of it as a metaphor to represent the social impact current lifestyle trends have on society. I think of it as the perfect explanation for the emergence of Type 2 diabetes, especially among children.

That day we talked about the growing trend of decreasing activity on playgrounds throughout the United States. We discussed the importance of role-modeling, and the fact that many kids rarely engage in physical play because their parents rarely do. After that I began watching the dynamics of park activity when I was at the neighborhood park with my three kids, Emily, Aaron, and Jordan.

Quite often – too often – as other children in the park are

playing, their parents are off on the side, talking on their cell phones or just sitting down. And they continue to be, regardless of the pleas of the kids to join them. Many times when I'm at a park, I will end up playing chase with those children as well as my own. After a while these parents who have pushed their kids off to play while they do something else look somewhat bewildered, realizing their kids are having a great time, but with someone else. It sometimes sparks a change, but for the most part, adults have forgotten how to play.

Nowadays, the message about activity is to some extent stifled by life's conveniences. Many times when you do see children on playgrounds, they've got some type of digital device with them. I love having PDAs, digital music players, and video games; they're part of today's world. But there's a time and a place for everything. These and other things, like endless television channels, are replacing physical activity. If you allow them to, they'll drag you and your children down. Make the decision that you will not allow your children or yourself to miss out on the significant and important benefits of exercise and regular activity. Don't let them miss out on the real joy that an active life provides.

There is plenty of evidence that staying active can help children mentally, too. In his book "Teaching with the Brain in Mind" (ASCD, 1998), author Eric Jensen writes: "Aerobic and other forms of 'toughening exercises' can have enduring mental benefits. The secret is that physical exercise alone appears to train a quick adrenaline-nonadrenaline response and rapid recovery. In other words, by working out your body, you'll better prepare your brain to respond to challenges rapidly. Moderate amounts of exercise, three times a week, 20 minutes a day, can have very beneficial effects."

We must guide our children, and provide them an example to follow. Among other things, their good health, and ours, depends on it.

MOST ADULTS WITH Type 2 diabetes seem to be in denial, whether they realize it or not. You are among them if you think you are overweight or it's difficult to lose weight because you have Type 2 diabetes. It's actually just the opposite. Most often, people have Type 2 diabetes because they've become inactive and overweight. Yes, other factors may contribute to the development of Type 2 diabetes. But don't be misled into thinking the primary causes are anything other than an extended waistline and a lack of consistent and vigorous activity.

To those who continue to underestimate or minimize the huge role poor weight management and a lack of regular exercise play in the occurrence of Type 2 diabetes, I quote the following bit of wisdom expressed by a noted cardiologist speaking at a medical conference I attended. "With heart disease," he told his audience, "and with Type 2 diabetes, genetics may load the gun, but inactivity and being overweight pulls the trigger."

He is not alone in this view. Many medical experts in the field of diabetes have proclaimed that most patients with Type 2 diabetes have acquired it as a BOS (Behaviorally Onset Syndrome), not as a traditional "disease." And, they add, "This population can reverse the condition if they so choose."

Yes, you read that last sentence correctly. Consistent and effective exercise coupled with intelligent weight loss and eating right can *reverse* the Type 2 condition in many people, as well as prevent it in almost all. Despite the physicians and some diabetes groups loudly proclaiming this amazing fact, however, most people with Type 2 are not even aware this possibility exists.

A simple explanation of a receptor's function is that it helps insulin transport glucose into the cells from the blood. The wrong food, too much food, and inactivity combine to elevate blood glucose levels in an overweight person. This, in turn results in the release of more insulin than normally produced. And those recurring "overdoses" of insulin can lead to a condition called hyperinsulinemia (over production of insulin), which over time causes damage to the endothelial cells. These cells protect your blood vessels. When they are damaged, you open yourself up to all the associated cardiovascular risks: arteriosclerosis, stroke, heart disease, etc.

Fortunately it isn't a permanent condition, or doesn't have to be. It's up to you. Are you willing to make the effort?

Antidote Reminder

**An exercise program improves
whole-body insulin sensitivity,
whole-body glucose metabolism,
and post-meal hyperglycemia.**

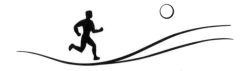

3

Empowering yourself

*'. . . if you make the decision yourself,
if you say, "This is something I want
to do," then it becomes something
you personally own.'*

EVER SINCE I can remember, I was consumed with becoming a champion at something. I admired anyone who excelled in his or her chosen field – athletes, speakers, leaders and actors, most of all. It wasn't just their performances and accomplishments I wanted to emulate. It was their confident attitude, as well.

I had a pretty typical upbringing as a child. My dad, an Irish New Yorker, was a lieutenant colonel in the Korean War. I didn't find out until I was older, but he received a Bronze Star for bravery. He didn't talk about it and didn't really want any praise or recognition for what he did. A bunker was under attack and he pulled a couple of guys out of the way of a mortar, and took a piece of shrapnel in his chin.

After his military service, he worked as an oceanographer and physicist for a division of NASA, the National Aviation and Space Administration. I loved hearing his stories of the sea creatures he and his co-workers encountered. It made me want to explore the wild, too. Probably the best trait I learned from my dad was a strong work ethic. He took only two sick days in his thirty-five years with NASA.

My mother is a first generation American Italian, short-tempered but loving. She was the only child of five in her family born in the U.S.A, and grew up in the steel towns of

Pennsylvania. One of the qualities she passed on to me was determination. When committed to a task, she is the type whose fingers cannot be pried from it until it is completed. After I was diagnosed with diabetes, my older brother Brian felt like he was pushed to the sidelines in terms of getting attention from our mom and dad. Just as it is for any kid with a disease, the attention was a mixed blessing for me. At times the consideration is nice, but you become aware that the attention is based on what's wrong with you instead of something positive you've done. You're trying to deflect the concern, but you're getting all the attention, and that's all your sibling sees.

Brian didn't like it, and let me know with simple kid tricks, like dropping me in the clothes dryer and turning it on. It was only for a couple of turns; two bounces and then he he'd let me out. If I hadn't been so skinny, I wouldn't have fit. (I also remember how protective of me Brian was whenever another neighborhood kid would make fun of me, or if I was having a BG problem.)

Unfortunately, my dad began to pull away from me. In part I think it was due to him being a scientist and being accustomed to analyzing the problem and finding a solution. Seeing your kid getting evacuated by ambulance every other weekend is a far more complex problem. It was difficult for him because he wasn't able to resolve the problems I was having with the management of my diabetes, and I was becoming more introverted in response to those problems.

I was the smallest kid in class, and a lot of the other kids pushed me around. I was a freak, a broken kid. I felt like rejected and defective merchandise, and I vowed that someday I would destroy the weakling I was. I knew I needed to

do something to change myself. I just didn't know what.
Then I found an old picture Bible.

I began leafing through the stories, and there, with one
of them, I saw a picture of what I desperately wanted to be.
It was a painting of Samson. He had muscles I had never
seen before, incredibly huge shoulders, giant arms and
veins that were bulging everywhere. He had a full-grown lion
in a headlock. I became transfixed with the image of strength
and power that he possessed.

That night I read, over and over, the full story about
Samson's conquests of the Philistines. Even though I understood only a small part of it, I was consumed with his power
and glorious strength. For probably the first time I prayed –
sincerely – that God would make me like Samson. I bar-
gained that if He did, I'd kill all the lions and Philistines He
wanted me to. I dreamed every day about being like Samson,
slaying lions if they crossed my path and saving other weakling people just like me.

The instant requests brought no changes, but it didn't
matter. This was a matter of need. Surely God would transform me if I pulled the right strings or said the right prayers.
This was my way to get out of the miserable existence I had
known. I was committed to change.

AS A PROFESSIONAL trainer, I have advised virtually every
type of person imaginable – from Olympic sprinters and pro
football players to juvenile delinquents, from early teens to
people in their nineties, from people worth hundreds of millions of dollars to people just getting by. They all share a common thread: Their success or failure at achieving their personal fitness goals depends on the goals *they* set for them-

selves, not on the goals I or anyone else set for them. Setting their own goals establishes them to some extent as the director of their destiny, and creates a level of commitment they can use to reach or exceed these goals. You've probably heard the saying, "If you don't make a decision, one will be made for you." It's correct.

I usually see a client for an hour per session, a minimum of twice a week. I always tell a new client, I'll show you how, but it's up to you. You have to make the decision yourself. Getting in shape needs to be an extension of your life. It's much easier to convince someone who has succeeded in some fashion before, because they understand that to succeed, you have to first establish the goal. It's building on past experience, so it's much easier for them to conceptualize what I'm telling them. You cannot "hit the mark" if the mark has not been set, right?

That's the key to personal fitness. It has to be something you *want* to do. That is Number One. It's about *your* decision, and not about someone twisting your arm into doing something you don't want to do. If it's done from a negative sense, because you "have to," you'll attempt to do it, but begrudgingly. You won't want to do it. You'll initially try to, but it won't be set in your heart to finish, and chances are you will not finish.

Likewise, if you do it out of fear or a sense of guilt because your wife's telling you to do it, or your husband or your mother or your father is telling you to do it, in essence you don't really want to do it. I know. I've been there. However, if you make the decision yourself, if you say, "This is something I want to do, and I'm going to do it! I'm going to look better. I'm going to feel better. I'm going to function bet-

ter. I'm going to help other people." Whatever the reason
might be, you then personally own the decision. It empow-
ers you to find a way to do it. And then it becomes something that becomes self-sustaining. It's driven from within.
That's why I say the very first, and most imperative, piece of
advice I can give to anyone is to set their own goals and clar-
ify their decision.

You don't have to aspire to be a champion. What is your
desire? If your desire is to lose 20 pounds, so be it; that's
fine. If your desire is to lose 100 pounds, so be it. If your
desire is to GAIN 20 pounds, because you're too thin (as I
once was), or if your desire is simply to engage in activity
three times a week because at present you do nothing, that's
all beautiful! It's all about your desire.

That's the "Exercise Prescription." It's not a single set of
exercises or a single specific routine. It's not "run this fast,
this far or for this long." And it's not "use this particular
device or piece of equipment," or "lift this much weight this
many times." Instead, it's your desire, and your decision to
realize that desire. For that reason, "The Exercise
Prescription" is not the same for everyone; not at all. It's
about showing you the light, and about you seeing it, about
seeing how much exercise benefits your life and then deciding to take advantage of it. Especially if you have diabetes or
you are a candidate to develop Type 2. It's never about
someone twisting your arm into doing something you don't
want to do.

WHEN SOMEONE COMES to me to work with them, the first
thing I want to establish – before I can tell them what to do
– is what they are trying to accomplish. Most often, they

don't know. It's a foggy concept, murky, with self-doubt. It's the biggest mistake people make when they decide to do something about their personal fitness. Because if your personal decision isn't clear, it doesn't resonate within your mind or heart.

A lot of people make a broad decision, like "I want to lose weight." It means absolutely nothing to the brain. As an attorney would say, it's vague and ambiguous. On the other side, if you step out and say to a friend, "I'm going to lose *ten* pounds by February 15," suddenly: "Click!" Psychologically, you've put yourself out there and it becomes a different game altogether.

When you start training, that statement keeps resonating in the brain. It forces you to comply with it, and you come up with one of two outcomes. Either you meet the goal, or you run away from it entirely. But you don't get the chance to be ambivalent about it. Being specific about your goal forces a compliance of sorts within you.

I once worked with an Italian guy, Joey. He was an incredible chef with his own cooking show on television. When he first came to me, he weighed 290 pounds, at 5 feet 7 inches. His torso was so big he could hold his arms out, and they looked like they were resting on a table. He was immense and fat, and he knew it.

As a chef he was always on the go, and now it was becoming more difficult for him to move around, because he had gotten so large. He loved being a chef, and knew how to make some of the best dishes imaginable. And like any good chef, he liked to taste what he'd made. He was around food all the time.

Joey became horrified with how big he had become.

The key is that he admitted it and was determined to make a change. I could have trained him all I wanted, but without the decision he made – without his personal resolve – he wouldn't have gotten there. He was incredibly disciplined.

In less than a year's time, Joey lost 101 pounds! The change was so drastic that, when he made his yearly tour through Italy and to a small town in France, some of his friends at a party he attended did not recognize him, at all. Even after speaking to them for ten minutes, they remarked, "You remind us so much of someone we know from the States." You can imagine his pride when he stopped them and laughingly said, "Guys, it's me, Joe!" He could not have been happier.

He had this vision that this is what he was going to do. He was going to do it regardless. And he did!

Most people, if they could look at their personal situation on a spreadsheet and see the benefits and the problems associated with their situation, would choose to take action. You can look better, or you can look worse. You can feel better, or you can feel worse. You can impress and motivate people, or you can just get by. For a person with diabetes, your A1c's are better, or they're worse; all the way down the line – your eyes, kidneys, circulatory system, heart – everything. (Hemoglobin A1c is a measurement that reflects average blood glucose for the last 60 to 90 days)

Everybody naturally would choose to feel better, to look better. Nobody sets out to feel worse; nobody sets out to look worse. But habits sometimes are very hard to break. It has to be a resolution that is not only definitive, but also firmly established. *"I will do this!* And I don't care what obstacles will come up." Because, mark my words, obstacles will present themselves, one way or another. They will come up.

When your decision is clear, though, it becomes much easier to see them just as obstacles, instead of excuses not to keep following through until you have achieved the goal you set for yourself. Remember, the decision is yours alone to make, and "If you don't make a decision, one will be made for you."

Antidote Reminder

Give yourself some freedom to make mistakes on the way to your goals. But remember: The only loser is the one who never tried. Pick an activity you like!

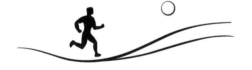

4

Finding a way

'You are never too old, too sick or too busy to get in shape. Those are just excuses that call out to everyone with diabetes, every day.'

NASA MOVED THE department that my father worked in, along with the Space Shuttle testing site, to the deep woods of Mississippi when I was 12. Due in part to the bad experiences I had had while living in Washington, DC, moving to a new place was great news to me. I thought I had it all figured out. I was a fan of the Tarzan television series, and the few pictures I had seen of the swamps in Mississippi looked like the Amazon where Tarzan lived. I figured the swamps there must be filled with huge snakes and crocodiles, too. And since the people in Mississippi couldn't possibly drive cars in the rainforest, I would have to paddle a canoe to school just like the native kids must do.

I pictured my new life with passion. This was going to be a great change, and I was ready. It took a few days to drive there. After much anticipation, we finally arrived. I was incredibly disappointed. Where was the quicksand, the jungle, and the gators and anacondas? "What are these cars doing here?" I asked myself. I was sincerely crushed when I discovered there were roads and buildings and regular people. It was a wake-up call to my naiveté, but within a short time I recovered and ended up loving the place. The kids there accepted me, regardless of my funny appearance.

I had gotten better with my eating habits and at managing my insulin, and was beginning to get more stable with my blood sugar levels. When I was well I spent most of my time in the outdoors, hunting in the woods, catching snakes, hiking, and diving from the railroad trestles into the Wolf River. One day I found a muscle magazine called *Ironman*, and became locked into the image I saw on the cover. It was a picture of an incredibly powerful athlete from Louisiana named Casey Viator.

This guy was a phenomenal strength athlete – a living version of Samson, the same huge arms, huge chest and huge deltoids. He had won the Mr. America championship while he was still a teenager. At 19, he was the youngest winner ever. He was bench pressing over 500 pounds for repetitions; squatting 700 pounds, and curling 300 pounds! Though I still thought about Samson, this wasn't just a painting in the Bible. Here was a real person, still alive, and he had the physique I wanted and needed.

Inside the *Ironman* magazine I saw all these pictures of exercises. I'm sitting there, as a kid, thinking, "How can I do this?" I mean, we're living in the boondocks of Mississippi. Even though there were no gyms near me at the time, I was convinced this was my solution that God had sent. He answered my prayer with that picture of Casey and that magazine, and I simply had to improvise.

I decided I would try to replicate what I saw in the *Ironman* magazine. I found a scrap steel yard that was maybe a half-mile from our house. I went there and asked the guys, "Hey, do you have any steel bars I could use?" And they said, "Yeah, there's some scrap stuff over there." I asked if it was okay if I took some things home, and they let me have three different bars.

Then I found this abandoned crane. The thing was all rusty and dilapidated, but I saw that it had these huge pulleys. It was very tall, and cables ran through it. I enlisted my two best friends, Ricky Greenwald and Frank Kish, and we shinnied up to the top of the crane. We sat there, day after day for hours, trying to knock the cotter pins out with hammers and screwdrivers. Ricky was half Iroquois Indian and Franky half Hungarian. I was half Italian and Irish. I became part Iroquois and part Hungarian, too, through the blood brother ritual we carried out in case one of us fell off the crane. The wonder wasn't that we never fell. It was that none of us developed tetanus from my rusty knife!

Finally we succeeded. We got a bunch of plates that were 25 pounds apiece. I'll never forget them: solid brass inside, steel on the outside, holes throughout. They were perfect.

We also raided construction sites at night, and "borrowed" the lumber we needed for the bench. We dragged off some cement and put it in buckets to make weights. We put together all this rickety equipment based on the exercises we saw in the magazine. We actually did a great job of building a makeshift gym in the tool shed in my backyard. We didn't spend a penny making our virtual gym. I couldn't have done it without the assistance of my "Huck Finn" friends.

THE MORAL OF this story, of course, is "Where there's a will, there's a way." Just because a gym isn't around the corner, or you don't have the finances to use a gym, that's no excuse. You can find something, somehow, some way – a park, a trail, a pool. You don't have to be thwarted by a lack of equipment or money. You can find things that will help you. There are plenty of opportunities in contemporary life

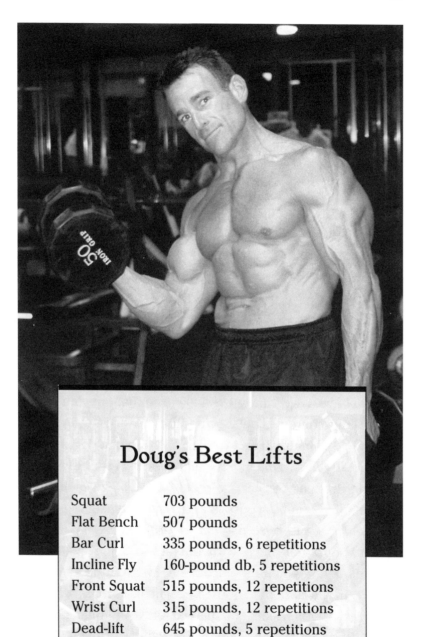

Doug's Best Lifts

Squat	703 pounds
Flat Bench	507 pounds
Bar Curl	335 pounds, 6 repetitions
Incline Fly	160-pound db, 5 repetitions
Front Squat	515 pounds, 12 repetitions
Wrist Curl	315 pounds, 12 repetitions
Dead-lift	645 pounds, 5 repetitions

and in the contemporary home.

Let's say you can't do a pushup. Not one. I bet you could do one leaning against a wall, and I bet if you did that for a week, you could move it down to a countertop, and then down to a stool. And within a month or two if you are patient and persistent, you'll be down on the floor, banging out pushups – even though you could not do even one when you started.

Without a doubt there are ways to exercise at home. You just have to be imaginative. Be willing, and you will find a way to improvise, a way to make it work. It's imperative to winning, to succeeding, to progressing. Because if you just follow everybody else, you're just going to get what they have. You have to be willing to step out on a limb and try something. If it doesn't work, fine; at least you know it doesn't and you are free to move on.

I'M SURE YOU'VE asked, "Why me? Why do I have diabetes?" I know I have. I don't have the answer to that one, but my little girl once told me, out of the blue: "Daddy, God doesn't make junk." And it's true. You are not less of a person or of poor quality because you have diabetes. If anything, you can become stronger. You can overcome the challenges diabetes presents if you apply yourself and simply refuse to give up.

Some of the best players in professional sports are from backgrounds filled with obstacles. Some even overcame diabetes. Among them: Jay Leeuwenburg played nine seasons in the National Football League. Before that, he was a college All-American and played on a national championship team at the University of Colorado. Chris Dudley had a long pro basketball career and has gone on to establish a national basketball camp for kids with diabetes. Adam

Morrison was a first-round draft choice in the National Basketball Association after leading the nation in scoring his senior season at Gonzaga; Gary Hall became a medal-winning Olympic swimmer; and Jonathan Hayes was one of the best tight ends in pro football when he played for the Kansas City Chiefs.

I know that at times life can present obstacles that seem insurmountable, and many diabetics experience frustration, depression and anger as they struggle to gain control of their disease. A sure way for us to fail is to adopt the "I am a victim" mentality. It is one of the most dangerous conditions someone with diabetes can encounter. It is what flavors our desire to blame others for our shortcomings, and it is a sure way to excuse yourself from doing anything good in life. We must overcome the obstacles life presents and push forward, for ourselves and for the ones counting on us.

Success, in any endeavor, isn't something that just happens. The committed make it happen regardless of circumstances. They have a tenacious spirit. That's what you must have when it comes to using exercise and physical conditioning to combat diabetes. You are never too old, too sick, or too busy to get in shape. Those are just excuses that call out to everyone with diabetes, every day. But they'll only bite those who respond.

I know the pitfalls. Too busy and too much to do? You'll get to it tomorrow? Reject that attitude like you would the plague. Some of the busiest people in America always figure out a way to squeeze in the things that are most important. That's why finding time to be active is almost always on the executive's daily schedule. Learn from them, especially if you have diabetes or are predisposed to develop Type 2.

Finding time can include climbing a few flights of stairs five or six or eight times a day at work, instead of riding the elevator. A brisk walk for 20 or 30 minutes every day at lunchtime can be part of it, too. If you play golf, park the cart and walk the course. If you cut your grass, jog behind the mower.

It is easy to fall into the "I am a victim" way of thinking. It is human nature to feel sorry for ourselves, to look for someone or some thing to blame for our adversity. But that doesn't make it wise, right, or helpful to either your health or success in life. I know that circumstances can seem to be overwhelming. If you want to "win" at whatever you're trying to do, though, you must be willing to step over the obstacles you have in your way, including negative feelings. You have to deal with your situation the best way you can. We all do.

Believe me, you will succeed even if you are dirt poor or feeling broken, worthless or unimportant – if you want it badly enough. I know, because I did.

Antidote Reminder

**It's okay to feel discouraged.
At one time or other, everyone with
diabetes has. But when obstacles arise, dedicate
yourself to overcoming them. Don't give up!**

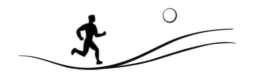

5

No magic potions

'. . . dietary "breakthroughs" and
weight-loss supplements that help
burn carbs are feeding on Americans'
laziness and naiveté.'

HOW MANY TIMES have you heard it said that getting in shape is about diet and exercise?   Thousands, probably. Well, this may surprise you, but I disagree. True fitness is not about diet and exercise. It's about exercise, first, and then diet.

Yes, they go together. But here in America, we have been fed so much propaganda about *this* new diet and *that* new weight-loss supplement that too many people have been led to believe that losing weight is all that matters, and that all it takes is some pill or fad program. Many jump from diet to diet, and eventually give up because nothing seems to work, or if it does at first, it doesn't last.

If you look closely at all of the books that require hundreds of pages to explain nutritional theories, suggest menus and provide recipes, most of them offer completely opposite viewpoints yet all claim to have found the secret breakthrough. The debate at the water cooler goes like this:

"It's low carb and high fat!"

"No, it's low fat and high carb!"

"I heard high protein, low-fat is the best."

"I'm on the South Beach diet, and it's great."

"I like Atkins myself. It really works!"

"Nah, the Mediterranean is the best."

The drawback to all of them is that they are "diets." They're something you're going to do for six weeks, or three months, or whatever. And after that? Typically it's, "I don't know what I'm going to do. I've reached my goal, and I'm going to go back and do . . . whatever." And that's the problem. People get talked into a short-term fix instead of changing the way they are living.

Many times I have had the same experience with clients. They leave for a couple years, and then come back. And almost the first thing they say is, "I know. I know. You told me not to just do the diet thing." They're coming back 50 pounds heavier. I tell them, "I wasn't telling you that just to keep your business." They are like a guy I know who has dieted seriously three or four times through his life. Each time he has lost more than 20 pounds, and for a time looked great. But within a year or two, he was ready for another diet, because diets only work as long as you stick to them. And no one can, or does, forever.

It's much easier to jump on a program than to moderate your lifestyle, but moderating your eating habits and making good choices about your daily diet is what's going to bring you that long-term success. A "diet" implies you're going to do something for a while, then get off it. Your *diet* describes the combination of food choices that comprises your day-to-day eating habits.

For me, diet doesn't have a fasting or denial component. It's a restructuring of not only *what* I eat, but also *how often* and *how much*. To get leaner and stronger, athletes break their eating patterns into smaller meals. By eating smaller meals you continually stimulate your metabolism to burn at a faster rate, and that helps you feel hungry less often. Eating big meals a couple times a day is a sure way to get your fat cells to expand and your waist to enlarge. Many people consistently eat far more food than they need.

To get in better or great shape, you also must pay attention to both the number of calories you take in and the types. You could compose a diet of 2,000 calories consisting of cake, candy, doughnuts, potato chips and regular soda, with an occasional burger. Or you could compose a diet of 2,000 calories consisting of ahi tuna, chicken breast, salad, broccoli, eggs, oatmeal, Granny Smith apples, almonds, and non-fat milk. Both have the same amount of calories, but they are worlds apart, aren't they!

The second 2,000-calorie diet includes food high in protein. The first has way too many carbohydrates and too much saturated fat. Protein is imperative in your diet because it is the building block for your tissue repair. I find it also helps dissipate my desire to eat more. The push for "fat-free" foods came about in the '80s. And what took fat's place? Carbohydrates. Not whole grain foods, but refined and thoroughly processed carbohydrates. That surge is one of the main reasons the obese and Type 2 diabetes populations have exploded.

None of this is meant to say you can never allow a little fun in your eating pattern. Even with an emphasis on eating the right foods and paying attention to the basic "balanced diet" that's been touted for decades, one day of the week I have whatever I want. Not every weekend, but often. I don't go hog wild, but I give myself some freedom.

By allowing that freedom, you haven't made things forbidden. Because if you make something forbidden, that's the apple you're going to end up concentrating on and end up picking. If you can't have it, it becomes exactly what you want. I'm a prime example. If I see a sign that says "Wet Paint," I have to touch to see if it's still wet. Or if I walk past a sign that reads, "Keep Off The Grass," like a kid, I have to put my foot on the grass. Following a healthy diet is no different. If you try to forbid certain foods, they are the ones you will most want. And you'll struggle with yourself over them, either because you gave in or because you want to.

The truth is, dietary "breakthroughs" and weight-loss supplements that help burn carbs or suppress appetites are feeding on Americans' laziness and naiveté. Those who believe that any of these can "transform your body into a lean fitness machine in only a few weeks," as the sales pitches claim, are buying into what I call the "Magic Potion Myth." They forget that they've been inactive for the last three years (or longer) and are 30 or 50 pounds overweight.

So why do we buy these products? Because they are supposedly quick, painless and external. How much effort is required, anyway, to put a pill in your mouth? But don't be deluded. If you tested every one of these supplements, diets and weight loss approaches, instead of just believing the hype and buying into them, you'd end up throwing most of them away. It took years to get out of shape; it will take a little time to reverse it. And why should weight loss be the primary solution?

Ultimately it boils down to this: You can feed somebody the best food they can get, but if they sit on the sofa all day long, every day, and do nothing, they'll still look, and be, out of shape. At the other end of the spectrum is the person you feed junk food to all the time but is out on the track every day. You do that for a couple months, then determine the overall health and fitness of those two people. The one who's been eating all the perfect foods but was not active is going to get smoked by the person who was eating bad food but stayed active.

Obviously, the ideal scenario is to combine both. To do the most for your health, you must combine the activities you like with good eating. But make no mistake about which one is first. When you combine good exercise along with good dietary practices, the positive effects on your body, health and diabetes produces results you didn't even think were possible.

MORE THAN ANYTHING else, your training program will influence your success at achieving the physical changes you desire. This I can guarantee. Those who deny that proper exercise is the primary factor in improving and maintaining your health are usually trying to sell you one of those new diets, pills, or products.

Too many people are looking for a quick fix for anything and everything. If it isn't a product or a pill, they buy some new piece of magical equipment, and they buy it without any forethought as to what it is they want to do with it. They've been sold an idea that they're going to look like X if they have one of these new devices.

They're buying machinery they see on television or in a magazine – some new ab lounge, ab chair, elliptical or home weight setup – under the expectation that this product is going to fix them, when in fact it has nothing at all to do with the solution at hand. They're looking at exercise only in the way that equipment is being sold to them.

The real solution to your fitness or weight loss goals rests almost solely on how badly you want to accomplish them.

My advice is to be sure your goal is solid before you invest in whatever it is you're about to buy. Ninety percent of the time those pieces of equipment get banished to the balcony or the garage, or they get unloaded at a future garage sale. The person who bought that equipment in the first place was looking for quick results, and that simply didn't happen.

My main message is worth repeating: The real solution is the decision you make. After deciding to change, the next most important key to getting in shape is to set your personal goals clearly. You can own not one of those pieces of equipment, and you'll still find a way to accomplish your goal. You can get all the equipment you want – one of everything that's on the market – and it's not going to change you a bit unless you've made the decision to change and you have a clear goal that you want to accomplish. That's paramount to improving your physical condition. Without the decision and a specific goal, the change won't happen.

It's like a weekend golfer who reads the golf magazines and goes to the golf stores and pro shops, and looks at every new driver that comes along. He reads the ads and watches the commercials, and he buys that latest new driver because he wants to hit the ball farther and straighter than ever before. He's sure his game is going to improve, but never sets foot on the driving range. He doesn't want to practice; he just wants to play. When he gets out on the course, his drives haven't improved. The guy next to him is whacking the ball farther than he is – and with a cheap club!

The reality is obvious: It's not just the club.

Similarly, if you want to improve your health and fitness, lessen or get off your medications as a Type 2, or gain better

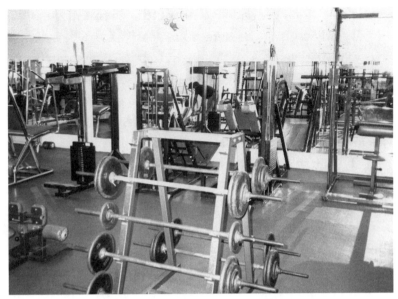

Doug's first "real" gym, in Biloxi.

control if you have Type 1, please avoid relying on "magic potions" and quick fixes. Find a reason that motivates you to change, a spark. This is not theory. It's the only reason I've won every title I've ever won. I set a goal for myself, and made the decision to do what it took to achieve it.

I realize that your goal probably is not to look as lean as a competitive sprinter, or as muscular as a bodybuilder. If it is, great! But if you're trying to manage your Type 1 diabetes or prevent Type 2, I hope you understand that the same principles will serve you just as well. The process in athletic conditioning and physique training, coupled with a sound dietary approach instead of fad diets and weight loss supplements, is absolutely flawless when it comes to reducing body fat and benefiting the body's cells, organs and circulatory system.

If you think about it, every one of those different diets and different programs claims to be the new solution. If that were really true, every advanced athlete, the ones who are winning, would be using and advocating those principles. We know what works and what doesn't. Rejecting the "Magic Potion Myths" and making a commitment to a sustained exercise program will help you win your fitness and weight-loss battles – regardless of past failures.

Antidote Reminder

A balanced diet is the best diet. Just eat the recommended number of servings for each food group every day. You won't need gimmicks to control weight or blood sugar.

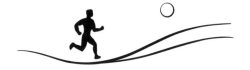

6

The best medicine

'The significance for a Type 1 should be clear . . . If you're not very active, even though you have your insulin regulated, you're not helping yourself.'

I BEGAN RESEARCHING the relationship of fitness to diabetes shortly after my first victories in powerlifting. After
five or so unsuccessful attempts, I won the Biloxi Bench
Press Championships, and then, a few months later, the Gulf
Coast Powerlifting Championships in Gulfport. I was incredibly elated after both victories. I wanted to understand the
effects that exercise and fitness had on a diabetic, not for
the medical benefits they might provide but strictly for self-
serving purposes. I did it to improve my performance and
my ability to win in strength competitions. I knew that exercise was "good for you physically," but that was secondary
to my drive to win.

Later, when I saw how consistently my medication levels dropped and how much my A1c's improved, it spurred
me to research the medical side to understand why these
events occurred. I began searching out anyone who could
explain the interactions surrounding a muscle cell's uptake
of amino acid and its relation to blood glucose levels.

I wanted to understand the biomechanics of cellular
changes as they related to exercise; why these changes were
for the better, and how to amplify the processes. In the
beginning I most commonly communicated with physicians,
chemists – even microbiologists – in social settings. They'd

ask me how to lose weight or strengthen their abdomen. After answering, I'd return questions about glucose uptake or protein assimilation. I think they found my questions both intriguing and amusing.

I studied pathology at the University of Southern Mississippi, due in part to an instructor I had met there. I can still picture his office, with his desk, a skeleton sitting in a chair, and a "Footprints" plaque on the wall. He was a very thoughtful and sincere educator, who asked me many questions about both my fitness and my thoughts about disease in general, since I had one. He taught me that knowledge and success are acquired in part as a result of a person's curiosity, their willingness to step out of the box and explore.

Now, I want to help you understand why physical fitness is some of the best medicine you can find to treat your disease.

A GOOD PLACE to start is with the term itself, and an examination of key components.

When you think of the word "fit," what comes to mind? Is it an image? A piece of equipment? Is it a look, a certain appearance? Or do you think of a condition, a person's physical ability to handle different types or certain amounts of activity? I'm afraid that too many people associate fitness with "handsome" or "attractive" or "just the right weight." The old saying that "Looks are deceiving." has never been more accurate than when applied to a person's level of fitness. I've trained some bigger people who looked "heavy" but had incredibly healthy hearts and bodies, and I've trained others who looked "thin" but were far from fit. Not everyone has the same body structure, so don't be deceived into thinking you have to be "skinny" to be fit. There are three basic body types:

> **mesomorphs** (primarily muscular with medium
> bone structure);
> **ectomorphs** (primarily skinny and usually with
> quick metabolism); and
> **endomorphs** (heavier bone structure with
> moderate to high body fat levels).

Don't get upset if at present you look far from the person you want to look like. You must understand that fitness is a physical state that will vary from person to person. Work with the structure you have; improve upon it instead of lamenting about how other people are "better off" than you. I wasted a good deal of energy feeling like I'd been "ripped off" in the genetics department, and it wasn't until I said, "I will win, regardless," that I actually did. Everyone has a cross of some sort to bear. To succeed, we have to work with what we have.

The President's Council on Physical Fitness has identified five dimensions to fitness that provide a great basis for evaluating your current physical condition. They include:

> **cardiorespiratory endurance** (the ability to
> deliver oxygen and nutrients to tissues and to
> remove wastes for sustained lengths of time);
> **muscular strength** (the ability to exert force for
> brief intervals);
> **muscular endurance** (the ability of a muscle or
> muscle group to sustain repetition in
> resistance activity);

flexibility (the ability of joints and muscles to
function through a full range of motion); and
body composition (frequently referred to as
Body Mass Index or BMI, which looks at
body fat versus lean body mass, i.e. bone,
muscle and organs).

The ideal workout program includes some type of activity that will help you improve all five aspects of fitness. There are two primary types of exercise you can utilize in your routine: *aerobic* (also called *cardiovascular)* and *anaerobic*. Aerobic tells you what it is; it requires oxygen. Cardiovascular tells you what it does; it works on the heart and vascular system. Swimming, running, brisk treadmill walking or jogging, cycling (whether riding a stationary bike or vigorously outdoors), cross-country skiing, soccer, and racquetball are examples of this type of exercise. Anaerobic is without oxygen; your muscles are firing on your stored fuel. It's resistance related, very short-term. A 40-yard sprint, for example, is not aerobic. Other examples of anaerobic exercise work are: using resistance machines, simple pushups and low to mid-rep weight lifting such as presses and curls with free weights.

Odd as it might seem, if I were forced to pick only one type of exercise for someone with diabetes, I would pick aerobic. The first 15 to 20 minutes of a workout is not aerobic. Your body's running on glycogen. After that short window of time and with your activity consistent, your body senses that this activity is going to go on for a while, so it shifts and begins converting body fat for use as a fuel. This is exactly what we want to happen. Instead of storing calories as fat, you're actively burning them. You're burning your body fat, and your metabolism gets a boost. Over time you become more physically and mentally capable of doing higher volumes and higher levels of activity. This causes the body to consume glucose on its own, and less insulin is required. This is the metabolic machine effect within your body that I referred to in Chapter 1.

MY OWN EXPERIENCE provides a great illustration of this. When I began training for the 2004 Mr. USA competition, it was after a difficult time. I was coming off a serious injury – six fractures to my lower right leg from a freak accident. It had required 13 screws to hold a plate between the tibia and fibula. I regained my strength pretty quickly, but aerobic work was much harder.

I charted my body weight, percentage of body fat, units of insulin per day, calories per day, and training activity. I had allowed my weight to climb to 228 pounds, and my body fat was relatively high at this weight, around 22 percent. I was taking in more than 5,000 calories per day, and since I'm a stickler for not getting "high," I was requiring more than a hundred units of insulin to cover it. At the outset I was doing about an hour of anaerobic work, heavy weights and fewer repetitions. Cardio was just starting.

Over the course of 20 weeks of training prior to winning the Mr. USA title, I increased my aerobic workout from nothing to 60 minutes, and maintained my anaerobic work at 90 minutes. These 90 minutes were increasingly fast-paced, almost to the point of no rest between sets. I reduced the amount of weight involved while increasing my repetitions. I trained four days a week in the beginning; added a fifth day after five

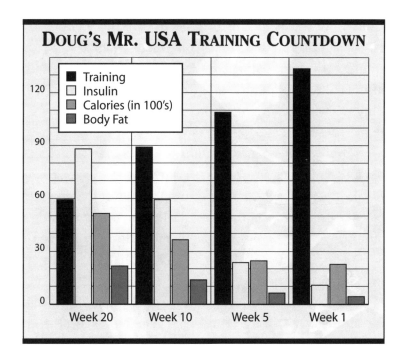

weeks, and a sixth after 12 weeks. The results were epic.

I entered the Mr. U.S.A. championships weighing only 187 pounds, and my body fat was down to 4.5 percent. In 20 weeks of intensive training I had lost 43 pounds; had reduced my body fat by about 17 percentage points; and most significantly, had lowered my insulin need by 90 percent! The reason? Persistent, intensive training, and, of course, the strong desire to do it.

THESE BENEFITS are available to everyone. It's a physiological pattern that applies to everyone, in varying degrees, depending on their desire, the amount of their activity, and their genetic makeup. Inactivity forces your Basal Metabolic Rate – the rate at which your body burns calories – to be slower than it was intended to be. Your BMR is going to sit there and not change. When you start engaging in serious training, however, especially when you activate the larger muscles like your quadriceps (frontal thigh), your gluteus or "glutes" (your rear end), and your hamstrings (back of thigh), your BMR starts increasing.

Initially, physicians thought this increase remained in effect just during the activity. During the exercise, your BMR is up, your heart rate is up, your blood pressure is up, everything is up. You've got all this stress coming on your body. The engine is using more fuel to go farther faster. The theory was that it remained that way for a little time afterward.

But over time, scientists were able to use more elaborate studies, and they found that a person's BMR didn't come up for just an hour, it came up for many hours afterwards. Sure it gradually returns to a basal level, but when you get into a system of consistent activity, not just once in a blue moon, your body becomes more capable, and your BMR starts elevating more easily and for longer periods of time.

On the other end of the spectrum, when someone is inactive and overeating, it can create that condition I referred to earlier, called hyperinsulinemia. That state of excess insulin is very damaging to the endothelial cells of the circulatory system. Even someone like me has to be careful. When I was lifting purely for strength, I weighed upwards of 240 pounds. I did little cardiovascular activity, and I was requiring so much insulin to transport the food I was eating that my sensitivity to insulin drastically dropped.

The significance for an inactive Type 1 should be clear. It's not enough to find that fine line balance for how much insulin you need based on your daily activity. If you're not very active, you're not helping yourself even though you have your insulin regulated. We were not designed to be inactive. Look at young children; they want to run and play, and they're designed to be active, not forever sitting. I'm not selling a diet program. I'm selling activity – activity for you and for the ones you love, plain and simple. Far better is the diabetic who is active but struggles to keep his or her sugars under control than the one who does nothing. Better physically, and better mentally.

PHYSICAL FITNESS is pivotal in another serious condition that closely resembles diabetes, and can be a harbinger of Type 2; it's called "insulin resistance." Unlike Type 1, in which the cells of the pancreas are not producing insulin, a person who is insulin resistant still produces insulin, actually overproducing it because his or her body is not efficiently utilizing the hormone. This also results in hyperinsulinemia and its related adverse impacts on the blood vessels and heart.

Dr. Gerald Reaven, professor emeritus in medicine at Stanford University, identified insulin resistance in 1968. Until then physicians believed the only issue was *how much* insulin the human body could produce. They didn't know that individuals vary greatly in their ability to *use* insulin, and were unaware that bodies that do not respond as well as they should to insulin try to compensate by producing *even more* insulin. This discovery helped to distinguish Type 2 as the condition that exists when a body is unable to produce enough extra insulin to overcome the malfunction of the cell receptors.

During a telephone interview with Louise Morrin, editor of the Canadian Association of Cardiac Rehabilitation newsletter, Dr. Reaven made a few statements that are worth repeating in a book that espouses exercise and fitness as *The Diabetes Antidote.*

"A regular exercise program, three or four days a week, for at least 30 minutes, will result in improved insulin sensitivity . . .

"Unequivocal metabolic benefits from exercise will not be achieved from a casual walk a couple nights a week. Significant, regular, chronic exercise is required to see improvements in insulin action . . . "

Are you starting to get the message? Are you wondering how to get started?

Antidote Reminder

Look for patterns in your blood sugar levels and your motivation levels based on the time of day that you exercise and the duration, intensity, and type of exercise.

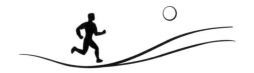

7

'My friend, Max'

'. . . the diet I suggest you follow is
different than anything you've heard
about. Eat breakfast like a king, lunch
like a prince, and dinner like a pauper.'

AFTER HEARING what I have to say about exercise and diabetes, a fellow came up to me and told me about a friend
who recently was diagnosed with Type 2 diabetes. His
friend's name, he told me, was Max. He wanted to know what
I would tell Max if he came to me for help. I don't know if
Max really exists, or if creating someone named Max was
just a way for this man to tell me about himself. Regardless,
it's a great way for me to give you an example of how everything you've read in this book so far can apply to you, to a
friend, or to a loved one.

Max is in his middle fifties. His first response to learning he has Type 2 was to become much more conscious of
what he eats. He has changed his diet without a precise
plan in mind. He's simply trying to eliminate the obvious
bad things. Our first conversation goes something like this:

"I just found out I have Type 2 diabetes, and I need your
help."

"Okay, Max. What is it you want to do?"

Max hesitates, as if he was expecting me to tell him
what to do, right on the spot.

"Well, I want to lose some weight. I want to lose 20
pounds."

"Okay. Twenty pounds is more than attainable. You can

definitely do it. When do you want to lose those 20 pounds?"

Max pauses again. He's being forced to think about this. Finally he admits, "I don't know."

"How much time can you devote to training," I ask, "be it with me or on your own? How much time are you willing to give to this?"

"How much time will it take?" Max fires back.

"That's up to you," I tell him. "If you can give me five days a week, it will take very little time. If you can only give me three days a week, it's going to take longer, but you'll still get there. Two days is a minimum."

Max moves into negotiation mode.

"For how long each day?"

"Let's say for an hour and a half. It's not going to be exhaustive, by any means," I tell him. "It'll start off at a half an hour; start off very, very slight, and then move it up. We'll keep moving it up. But I don't want to overload you, and get you so that you can't do anything."

I continue, explaining so that Max isn't overwhelmed.

"We'll ease into this, for two reasons. Number one, physically it's going to be too much for you if we go too fast. And number two, emotionally it'll seem insurmountable, and you'll end up rejecting it.

"But if you start off with just enough activity, it keeps feeding you, and you see a little bit of success. As soon as you see that success, you use it. Stick it in your mind: 'I did it! I lost two pounds. You know what! I can lose 20. I lost three pounds, five pounds – I can lose 20. I can lose 30!'

"Once that little bit of success is realized, the road is paved. You know you did it."

Max has something else on his mind. I can tell.

"I don't have an hour and a half," he says.

"Oh but Max, you do. Because if you don't, ten years from now, or maybe in just a few, you're going to have all the time you want, being spent on a dialysis unit. And you don't want that. It's much easier to arrest the problem now than to deal with the complications later."

MAX AND OTHERS like him need to know what's going on in their bodies. In either form, diabetes is known as the silent killer because people do not confront the disease until various functions in their bodies begin breaking down. It doesn't have to be that way. My goal is to show him – and you – how to turn diabetes, or being overweight and in a pre-Type 2 condition, into an *advantage*, before it takes control.

"If I lose 20 pounds," Max responds, "what's that going to do for my diabetes?"

"Chances are, if you're 20 or 30 over where you should be and you drop that extra weight, and have become very active, you'll get off your medication. You'll become un-diabetic."

Max hears this and looks at me as if he's beginning to think I'm a kook.

"It's much easier to do than people are led to believe," I continue, "far easier to do than people are led to believe, primarily through cardiovascular work. The cell receptor opens up greatly when there's a lot of cardiovascular work."

I offer myself as proof. "The perfect example," I tell Max, "is a physique competition. When I'm getting ready for a show, the amount of insulin that I require drops, drastically, as a result of the training I'm doing."

"My Type 2 is *reversible?*" Max gasps. He'd never heard that before.

"Yes. It's not as if your arm is on fire," I answer. "It's a very subtle and muted problem. It can be successfully treated with regular exercise to go along with weight loss."

"Which diet do you recommend I get on?" Max asks.

"I don't favor any particular diet," I answer quickly.

I can tell right away that Max was not expecting to hear that from me. To me it's more important to gauge *how much* you eat, what type of food you're eating, and *when* you eat it, rather than *what* you eat, which is what almost all diets focus on. It's very common in America to eat very large meals. We live in the land of the "bigger burger" and the "all-you-can-eat buffet" (which I used to get kicked out of pretty regularly). We eat a big meal, and then what? We go to sleep!

"Max," I say, "the diet I suggest you follow is different than anything you've read or heard about. It's this simple: Eat breakfast like a king, lunch like a prince, and dinner like a pauper. And drop your carbohydrate intake at dinner. For most people, it's breakfast like a pauper, if at all, and dinner like a king. But it ought to be the other way. If you do that, you'll use the calories you take in a whole lot more efficiently throughout each day. That will help you control your blood sugar, and when you exercise, you'll get more benefit from it."

By now, Max isn't quite sure what to say next. Or what to do. Finally, his true feelings come out.

"I'm just scared. I don't know what I want."

MOST PEOPLE WHO step into a fitness facility, or ask for advice, are a lot like Max. They may or may not have been diagnosed with Type 2, but over the years they have seen their health decline in some fashion, or their fitness decline. They've put on some weight; maybe it's come on gradually, or maybe it's come on suddenly. But they've noticed that they've declined. Their ability to get out and run for half a mile has become less and less. And they're aware of it.

It's a matter of them acknowledging the truth. They know the truth. It's a matter of them being willing to put on glasses and see it, admitting it to themselves. It doesn't matter how far off the mark you are. The important thing is, "What's the mark?" The mark is what's imperative.

You have to figure out where you want to go, what you want to accomplish, and the right way to get there. Think about it; the way to get to your goal is secondary to what that goal is. Because without defining what it is you're doing, you can figuratively get on every road you want, but you're not going anywhere. So with Max, I'm going to push back.

"Where is it you're going, Max? You want to go somewhere. You want to feel better. You want to look better. Right?"

"Yes."

"Everybody does, even athletes. They want to perform better. Right?"

"Yes."

Do they want to look better?"

"Sure."

"Do they want to feel better?"

"Yes."

"But again, even they have to be specific about where it is they're going with their exercise program. And why they're going there. You see the results. They improve, and they keep improving, and they are better because of it.

"Max, it's not my decision. It's your decision. You've made the decision that you want to change something, and that's a grand decision to make. Because it's going to benefit you. It's going to benefit your body. It's going to benefit your kidneys, your eyes, your circulatory system. It's going to benefit your entire body. It's going to benefit your kids. It's going to benefit your friends. It's going to benefit other people. You can end up becoming a leader for other people."

Max is thinking I might be getting a little carried away. "Just tell me what I should do," he says, a bit impatiently.

"It's very, very simple," I tell him. "You've done the right thing, the hardest thing. You've made the decision that you want to change, that you're going to change. You've made the decision to take responsibility for your health. So now it's a matter of defining that change, and sticking to the program to get there.

"It's easier said than done. I'll grant you that. But believe it or not, in most cases it's never said. But once it is said, once you've set a specific goal, it becomes easier to succeed. Now it's clear to you. It becomes, 'What's going to work best for me?'

"What do you like to do? Do you like to walk? Do you like to run? Did you swim? Did you hike? Did you ride a bike?"

"Believe it or not," Max says, patting his enlarged tummy, "I was a sprinter in high school. Ran some hurdles, too. I was actually pretty good, but you'd never know it now."

"Max, we mustn't concentrate on the picture we don't like, the one we don't want to be. In our minds we must see the picture we desire, the picture we want to achieve, and then strive for it. That's the way I've won every championship I've won."

Before Max can agree or disagree, I give him what I consider to be the keys to getting in shape. They are the factors I believe to be the antidote to diabetes and the antidote to failure. People succeed, I firmly believe, when they apply the following principles:

> **Faith** – You need only a small portion to take a chance and have a hope, a vision. You don't need status, or talent to apply it, and you're never too young or too old to start.
>
> **Purpose** – There has to be a reason you consider legitimate to lead you and help you get in shape. Not legitimate to me or to your friends. *To you.*
>
> **Wisdom** – That means choosing the things you believe are worthwhile endeavors.
>
> **Application** – It's all about honest, hard work.
>
> **Perseverance** – You must refuse to quit . . . regardless.

"So where do I start?" Max asks.

"You already have," I tell him. "Let's get out a calendar, and put down a date. We'll work back from that."

Antidote Reminder

**Try to find a friend to join you
in your endeavors, but if you are
not able to find a friend to join you,
succeed anyway!**

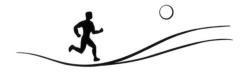

8

Words of caution

*'The point of The Diabetes Antidote
is to identify ways you can prevent
the medical complications of diabetes
with a regular exercise regimen.'*

I HAVE MANAGED to avoid the long-term health problems so common with diabetes. My feet, my eyes, my kidneys, and my circulatory system all are in good condition. And I expect them to remain so. But that's not to say I haven't had my share of challenges and lessons learned the hard way. The following story from my early years in powerlifting is a good example.

I was training at Keesler Air Force Base in Biloxi, Mississippi with a friend. We were training legs together. He could do an enormous amount of weight, and I could too – heavy leg presses up to 1,400 pounds and heavy squats, sets of eight to ten with 600 pounds. We were driving back from Biloxi after our workout, and I was up ahead. I pulled over because I could feel that I was getting low. I was trying to find something to eat because I forgot to replace the glucose in my bag.

The friend I was with pulled off behind me, and came over and said, "Doug, what's gong on?" I was dripping with sweat and at that point couldn't even speak. He knew I was diabetic, and he knew I needed help. This was before cell phones, but fortunately there was a pay phone nearby, so he was able to call the paramedics.

They loaded me onto a stretcher and took me to

Gulfport Memorial Hospital. The emergency room techs told me later that when I got there, my legs had started to undergo extreme cramping because I was strapped into the bed. My legs were exhausted from training and, due to electrolyte imbalances from the low sugar level, they began hyperextending. They said it sounded like my knees were cracking, and they could hear it even through my roaring in pain. My legs were literally lifting my body off the surface of the bed on my heels.

I have an extremely high pain threshold, but my legs felt as though they were slowly being broken in half. I was screaming, coming up out of the bed as the pain intensified, and pulling up on the straps. As you might imagine, one broke. As they wheeled me into the emergency room I was grabbing everything around me I could find. These techs were accustomed to treating insulin shock, but never on a strength athlete. At first they thought I was amped up on amphetamines.

At the time I was about 230 pounds, a big boy. An attractive young nurse told me later that she jumped on my chest in the ER to try to hold me down to attach an IV, and she said it was like a kid kicking a squirrel. I just threw her off. She was a bubbly little Southern girl, and jokingly told me later, in the sweetest accent, "You're the only man who ever kicked me off him in my whole life." I guess I should have asked for a second chance.

They had relocked my legs in, but my right arm was free. After I threw the nurse, the emergency room doctor came in to run the IV. He was trying to attach it in my left hand, as the other two techs held my torso down. The pretty nurse had bounced right back up and was trying to soothe me with a passive voice. And it worked until I felt this slight pricking sensation. I still had not received any glucose and was increasingly incoherent; I just felt this prick in my hand. I was told later that I reached over with eyes closed and, unfortunately, grabbed that doctor's hand. I crushed his wrist and metatarsals.

Two weeks later I was in a night club on a Saturday night. I'm talking to a girl up in the front, and I see a guy over in the corner, looking at me. He has a beard, and he's older; I'm twenty-two.

I nodded and kept on talking to the girl, Tina. I looked over again, and he was still staring at me, and I started wondering, "What's this guy looking at?" Then he started walking over toward me. I was thinking, "I've seen this face before; what's going on?"

He came over to me, and I saw that his arm was in a cast all the way up to his shoulder. I asked him, "Did I have something to do with this? Is this from the hospital?"

He said, "You don't remember me, do you?"

I looked at his arm, and I said, "Did I do that to you?"

He said yes, then told me the whole story. I felt terrible about it, but he said, "It's fine. It's fine. You gave me a ten-week paid vacation and the hand will be fine. Don't worry about it."

Following that, I went back to the hospital and apologized. I met everybody in the ER, and they all said, "Good God, we've never seen anything like that." That pretty nurse took me on a tour and told me what happened: "You pulled the curtains down here . . . You knocked the tables down over here." Along the way this guy came over, a big guy about 260 pounds. He said, "I remember you."

One of the nurses laughingly said to him, "Kevin, you deserted us all." He answered with his Southern drawl, "Hellllll no, he was 'bout to kill ya'll." Turning to me, he said, "after what you did to me I wasn't gonna deal with no more . . . helllll no"

This guy is a comedian repeating the "helllll no" line every chance he gets, and I'm laughing as I asked what happened next. He said, "I came up behind you, when you first came in, and I was in my shirt, pushing the bed. You reached back and grabbed my shirt with your hand and ripped my whole shirt off me . . . "

"Then what happened," I asked. The nurse jumped in and said, "I'll tell you what happened. Kevin says, 'Hellllll no, I ain't dealin' with this shit. I'll go an' get some coffee,' and he took off."

The point of the story, I guess you could say, is never let your sugar get too low. And never feel like you're the "only one."

IN ALL SERIOUSNESS, it would be irresponsible if this book did not acknowledge the risks associated with diabetes. It is a complicated and very serious medical condition that requires conscientious attention to many medical factors. But I want to make it clear: The point of *The Diabetes Antidote* is to address the methods of avoiding those risks, and the ways you can prevent those complications with a regular exercise regimen. It is up to you to not become a statistic, but here are some key points that should never be overlooked.

1. Consult with your physician before launching into an ambitious exercise program. Make sure your blood

pressure and cholesterol readings are within ranges
that are safe for the kind of activity you are planning.

2. Be sure you understand the relationship between your
    body's response to sustained aerobic exercise and its
    normal use of insulin. This is critical when it comes to
    regulating your insulin level before and after any exer-
    cise, and avoiding lows during your workout. Develop
    strategies regarding when you eat in relation to when
    you exercise; when you test your blood glucose; and
    the appropriate insulin dose prior to exercising.
    Always, keep with you some type of emergency food
    that is a ready source of glucose.

3. Learn to recognize the signs your body sends when you
    are experiencing low or high blood sugar. Being able to
    react quickly to the first symptoms of these conditions
    will help you avoid serious complications. Don't exer-
    cise alone. Make sure that someone nearby is aware
    that you have diabetes so that they are prepared to
    respond quickly and appropriately if you become dis-
    oriented or impaired.

4. Check your sugars regularly! At times we all think our
    blood glucose levels are okay – until we test. If you have
    Type 1 diabetes, be sure to check your blood glucose
    before *and after* physical activity, and do so until you are
    accustomed to its effect. Remember that exercise has
    an insulin-like effect on muscle glucose transport, and
    often results in a decrease in plasma glucose levels that
    persists during the post-exercise period.

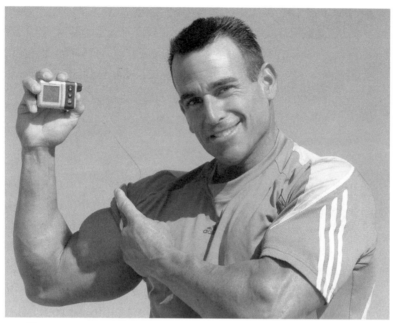

DOUG USES SEVERAL BLOOD GLUCOSE METERS IN HIS DAILY LIFE.

5. Use your blood glucose meter. Though it may seem like a labor, this is one of the most vital keys to prevention and safety. Every single winning athlete I know who has diabetes has developed a consistent and frequent practice of using their blood glucose meter. I have different meters throughout my daily life, in the car, in the gym bag, in my personal bag. The more frequently I check my BG levels, the easier it is to accomplish the training goals and avoid a potentially serious situation.

6. Keep in step with your feet. This begins with making sure you have the right shoes for your feet and good socks. If you are exercising in a way that taxes your feet, such as running, cycling, skiing or using a treadmill, stepper, or

elliptical, be sure to increase your intensity and time gradually so that you avoid blisters or other strain on the nerves in your feet. Check your feet; I do. Use lotions or other agents to avoid cracking. Obviously, if you experience numbness, itching, burning, or tingling, or if your feet are often cold when there's no normal reason for it, see your doctor.

7. Watch your eyes. If you have developed retinal hemorrhages or other symptoms of diabetic retinopathy, ask your physician which exercises are best for you to engage in. Anaerobic exercise, for example, almost always raises your blood pressure. You also should beware of activities that cause your body to bounce or change directions suddenly, such as jumping rope, and any that would cause pressure changes within your eyes, such as underwater diving, high mountain hiking, climbing or some skiing. Pass on exercise that causes your eyes to be below your heart, such as touching your toes.

8. Never drastically alter your exercise or medication or dietary habits! I'm all in favor of drastically altering your goals and planning for success, but use wisdom in your approach. You must, if you really want to succeed.

9. For either Type 1 or 2, "Self Talk" is imperative. You are not diseased; you are who you are. Sure, you carry a disease. But the disease doesn't carry you. You have incredible talents and opportunities; some that are evident and some still hidden. Explore your options and never give up!

10. If you are the parent of a child with diabetes, please realize the importance to your child of understanding, compassion and, yes, in some instances, tough love. For some parents it can become a difficult issue for the relationship between you and your child, and your spouse, too. Locate other parents who have children with diabetes. By working together you can alleviate your concerns; your child can make new friends; and you will empower each other. Children With Diabetes is hands-down the best resource I know for parents of children with diabetes.
Visit them at <u>www.childrenwithdiabetes.com</u>

THE STATISTICS ABOUT the increased health risks associated with diabetes used to scare the hell out of me when I was a child: "Eighty-five percent of diabetics will develop kidney failure. Your life expectancy is reduced by up to 30 percent. Your chances of heart disease is increased three-fold, and on and on."

Regarding those statistics, I remember a preacher friend from southern California – his name was Bob – who, when I told him about the statistical hype surrounding diabetes, told me: "Doug, the only statistic I know that is absolute is the death rate. It's 100 percent. Everyone dies. But how you live is up to you."

Truer words were never spoken. *You* decide if you become a diabetes statistic. No one else, and nothing else, does. Remember what I said earlier in this book. Make a decision, or one will be made for you. Use those statistics, if you like, as a goal to beat. It was one of my motivators.

If you have diabetes and your blood sugar levels were never out of control, would you be at any greater risk for heart disease, kidney failure or retinopathy? Absolutely not.

Antidote Reminder

If you have Type 1 diabetes, be sure to check your blood glucose levels before *and after* physical activity, and do so until you are accustomed to the effect it has on you.

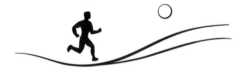

9

Mr. Universe

'Needless to say, I do not use, nor do I advocate using, any performance enhancing drugs. Their use is bad news – all the more so if you have diabetes.'

I PURSUED MY commitment to strength training and exercise with a Spartan passion. I did not care how painful the training was, how early I had to get up, or how hard I'd have to push myself. My goal to excel was firmly set, and I was relentless in accomplishing it. The results became obvious once I reached high school.

When I started playing football in the seventh grade, I was still one of the weaker kids on my team. But a couple years later I had become one of the strongest players on my high school team and soon after, one of the strongest in the nation. I was a pretty good running back – I won the most valuable running back award one year – but I loved hitting with a passion and actually preferred cornerback.

I had aspirations of playing college football when I enrolled at the University of Southern Mississippi. I had good speed and a load of hitting power from all the heavy bench pressing and squats. I quickly reached a crossroads, though. I had to decide if I was going to pursue football or strength shows, and it was a very difficult decision for me to make. I had started competing in powerlifting when I was 15 years old. My first show of strength was actually a competition of high school football players. I can still remember as our team drove to Gulfport in a bus and competed against

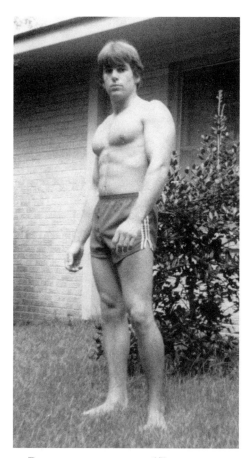

DOUG AS A MUSCULAR 17-YEAR-OLD.

the Gulfport and Biloxi teams. I didn't do that well but did have one of the best squats in that show. In my first legitimate powerlifting contest I did not even place, but knew that I would if I did not give up.

Although the coaches at Southern Mississippi pursued me to play football, I chose strength and stopped playing ball. I wanted to be the best in the nation at whichever I did. At the time, I thought if I continued with strength I would fol-

low Arnold Schwarzenegger's lead and become one of the
strongest men in the United States, make loads of money,
and have beautiful women hanging off me all the time.
Though I did become one of the strongest males in the U.S.
in my weight class, the other parts of the plan haven't
worked out the way I intended, at least not yet.

There were a number of renowned strength athletes on
the Gulf Coast. The owner of the gym where I trained was
"Doc" Rhodes, who had won the Pan American
Championships. Another was Vinson Keyhea, who became
one of my best friends. He was an incredible athlete, built for
strength. He went on to set world records in the deadlift.
With their help and encouragement, I went from being "the
bag of bones" to winner of six powerlifting championships,
in various classes from the 165-pound class all the way up to
the 242-pound class. I set university and state records, and
finally an American record.

The lifters from Biloxi had quite the reputation. You'd
hear wild stories about the competitors all the time – "This
guy Joey is an animal . . . I heard Kenny lifted the rear of a
van . . . I heard their heavyweight actually threw down a
bull!" . . . everything you can imagine. So you were nervous
as can be getting ready for one of these shows, especially
your first one. When you began to talk to the big guys at
these strength shows, the nervousness abated. Even though
the sport attracts the strongest men in the world, most are
incredibly kind and gracious, especially toward new and
younger lifters. They encourage you to do your best, and
when you hit your lifts or exceeded them, they joined you in
your elation. Standing on the winner's platform makes your
heart spin. Everything changes when you win. You're vali-

dated, uplifted, and feel like the conqueror. There is nothing that compares with the feeling of winning!

I SWITCHED FROM powerlifting to bodybuilding at the age of 20. I had done what I set out to do: set an American record in the bench press. This established me as the strongest in the nation for my weight class in what is considered the best test of upper body strength. Though I had first been inspired by pure strength, physical appearance was also vital to me. Physique wasn't a new thing for me – I had always aspired to look both "strong and fit." As a youth I attempted to excel in any form of exercise – sprinting, chin ups, push-ups, high jumps – anything that exemplified strength and physical prowess. Powerlifting had made me incredibly strong. Presses with hundreds of pounds, curls with 300 pounds, and even lifting the rear end of a car were now not that difficult. But as you might assume, it also came at a price. It was making me considerably slower, and maintaining that weight required copious amounts of food and insulin, which resulted in poor sensitivity to blood sugar fluctuations.

The two sports are very different. With powerlifting, it's all about strength. They don't care how little body fat or how much muscle you have. It's the 500-pound bench presses and the 700-pound squats that rule the day. With bodybuilding, it's all about body composition, which is a calculation of body fat versus lean body mass, i.e. bone, muscle and organs. So on the health side of things, physique competition is far healthier because of the requirement for low body fat and for fitness rather than pure strength.

Within a year and a half after I switched sports, I won the Mr. Southern U.S.A. Bodybuilding Championships. That got me an invitation to come to Los Angeles, and that was incredible! I was this naïve kid from Mississippi. I could tell you how to find an alligator or snapping turtle in a swamp, but I knew nothing about the faster sides of life. Landing in LA, I marveled at so many girls with colored hair, bright smiles and tanned bodies seemingly everywhere in the airport! I'd never seen anything like it. I began training at the famous Gold's and World's gyms in Venice and Santa Monica. All of a sudden, I was rubbing shoulders with the "stars" who came into those places, guys like Hulk Hogan, James Caan, Tony Curtis and, of course, the future governor of California, Arnold himself. I started appearing in the various muscle magazines I once idolized. I even appeared in a couple of television commercials.

After I met the movie star who became known as "The Terminator" for the character he played before turning to politics, my goal became winning Mr. Universe, just as he had. It took me years, but after more than a few setbacks (including a couple of near death run-ins, not medically related) stubbornness won out, and in November 2006, I did it!

THE APPROACH MOST bodybuilders follow is to build up muscle in between competitions, then reduce body fat while preserving muscle in the three to four months before a competition. That's the sequence I was referring to when I cited my experiences leading up to the Mr. U.S.A. contest in 2004. But that's not the practice I followed leading up to Mr. Universe. I have since learned that staying leaner year-round is not only less taxing for me physically, but it also makes it easier to manage my diabetes.

Building up muscle is a complex process of increasing

calories by sometimes as much as a thousand a day, eating more often each day, and choosing the mix of carbohydrates, protein, and fats that will achieve the chosen specific goals for muscular development. It also involves significant resistance weight training and vigorous cardiovascular training. For someone with diabetes, this presents some real challenges when it comes to managing what becomes a very delicate insulin balance under such conditions, as you can imagine.

To give an example, I had an abnormally difficult blood sugar day on the actual Mr. Universe contest day. The one day it needed to be perfect, it was anything but. This was the first time I had competed using a pump, and I was not thoroughly experienced with the extreme fluctuations I underwent without long-acting insulin in my system.

My total daily intake of insulin was down to only 10-15 units a day, a result of the extreme activity I was engaged in. However, by the morning of the show, I had not trained for four days straight. I had upped my basal dosage, but not enough. My blood glucose was elevated, and had been for some time. This isn't the best state for a physique competitor, because the dehydrating effects ruins the muscle's ability to properly function and pump up.

Notes I made that morning (obscenities removed) demonstrate just how tricky this process can be when diabetes is part of the equation:

Sugar was at 146 when I tested at 5:12 a.m. I took four units of Novolog for breakfast with two whole eggs plus five whites, three cups of oatmeal and black coffee. Took three multi mineral tabs plus some EFA's (essential fatty acids i.e. omega 3/etc.) along with a branched chain amino acid complex and a nitric oxide booster to prep for the event. All of these items I had been using prior to the event.

At 6:30 a.m. my sugar was stable, and I had some more slow burning carbohydrates but refrained from taking any more insulin to avoid a low. An hour and a half later, it had more than doubled, to 296!

Since I had completely stopped my aerobic activity on the Wednesday prior to the show, it was obvious that by Saturday morning my body had begun to miss the extreme expenditure it was accustomed to and was slow to respond even with all this extra insulin coming in. Add in the nervous energy I had for the event and the stress of trying to fix the situation, and the problem worsened. Those of you with Type 1 who have experienced this dilemma know how irritating it can be.

Half an hour later, my reading had dropped to only 196, which was still too high. I decided I needed activity, immediately so I ran some sprints, five sets of 50 yards. At 9:05 a.m. I was still at 191, so I took five units more of Novolog. By 10:23 a.m. my reading had finally dropped, to 119, but I had started cramping, badly in my hands in particular.

Regardless, I took in electrolytes, solved the problem and won the event. The rest of the day was far easier, and the night performance went very well. Friends from Los Angeles and northern California celebrated with me – right after I called my little ones and heard their shouts of joy. Nothing tops that.

THE EVENT ITSELF was spectacular; teams from all over the world with the UK, Canada and France having the best teams. The Friday night before the event I met a number of great people and began looking at the competitors. At this point in a contest the work has been done; it's almost a matter of going through the motions. I actually won the Mr. Universe 15 weeks before it started. If you are not "ready" on the show date, you can forget it. Just like with your goals, you set the goal and do the work; when the date comes it's simply a reiteration of the work you've already done. There were more than a few rugged competitors who showed up, one in particular from Canada and one from the U.K.

The night before, I also began looking to see if any "users" had shown up. As you probably know, the use of anabolic steroids is widespread in most professional sports, and "untested" strength and physique athletes are the leading users. Do not be misled into thinking this is a new issue. It isn't.

Indeed, when I first started lifting in California back in the mid-1980s, more than a few pro ballplayers were getting their drug advice and drugs from athletes I knew in the fitness world. The knowledge that some of these athletes and creative chemists had regarding what type of drugs to take surpassed most physicians' knowledge. These drugs are known by a variety of names: "Juice," "Sauce," "Roids," "Roidios," "PED's" (performance enhancing drugs), "Growth" (growth hormone), and their use is fairly rampant.

On the other hand, many professional athletes are clean, and these men and women deserve more credit than they receive.

Needless to say, I do not use, nor do I advocate using, any type of performance enhancing drugs. I still consider it a conquest whenever people at a gym I'm visiting or even at the competition would whisper, "Look at that guy. He's using . . . he's on drugs." It is a compliment in that to get to a level where you look like you are using drugs when in fact you are drug free, it means you have done your work very well.

The organizations within which I compete are 100 percent drug free. Everyone who competes in INBA and World Drug Free Powerlifting Federation-sanctioned events are tested through urinalysis and/or blood testing under the same guidelines as the International Olympic Committee. Every competitor must be completely "clean" to participate in natural powerlifting and physique competitions. A few guys failed the test in the Universe contest, and I'm happy the test is in place.

SINCE I KNOW it's of interest, I will elaborate a little bit on the aspects of drug use in sports. Anabolic agents and performance enhancing hormones mimic the hormone testosterone, which is the primary male hormone responsible for strength, aggression and recovery. It is the first and last element that athletes are interested in; these drugs help the body become strong by speeding up the repair of damaged tissue at a much higher than normal ratio. The difference between "natural" athletes and those using drugs is pretty pronounced. When someone compares a "natural athlete" to one using drugs, it means the "natural athlete" has brought his or her body to the upper levels of accomplishment. Those of us who have done this naturally share a great feeling.

I've helped some high schools develop their strength and conditioning programs for various athletic teams, and have been surprised at how many kids in the 10th to 12th grades knew where to get anabolic agents when I asked. Truth of the matter is that many times what they're getting access to are bogus drugs, total forgeries. The fake drug business is big business, and I'd assume more than half of the drugs being purchased underground are not real. And that makes them even more dangerous, in that if they aren't coming from a pharmaceutical company, then they're probably coming from Barney's bathtub.

Performance enhancing drug use is bad news, but all the more so if you have diabetes. I'm sure you have seen some of the problems associated with their usage, but it bears repeating: endocrine problems, cardiovascular issues including risk of heart attack and stroke, kidney damage, elevated blood pressure, risk of blood vessel hemorrhaging (something people with diabetes do not want), premature bone fusion, sterility, behavioral problems, (dependence, aggression), gynecomastia (female breast tissue growing on a male); and in females, reduced fertility rate, deeper voices, growth of facial hair, and behavioral changes, among other things.

One of my former clients had been the president of one of the most renowned biotech companies of our time. It was responsible for the development of DNA recombinant technology i.e. "human insulin." He and I, along with a geneticist who worked for him, were chatting about athletes' use of performance enhancing drugs and GH (growth hormone).

GH is literally a wonder hormone. It's the main reason young people look and behave young, and the declining rate of this hormone is one of the main contributors to the aging process. However, when athletes use drugs, they fall prey to the "more is better" syndrome, and this can be fatal. Something like growth hormone causes cellular growth – in all cells; so if you have cancerous cells, it spurs their growth too. Obviously, the use of GH is fine under a physician's advice; such use and its dosages are moderated. Many athletes who are using PED's are getting advice from some guy at the gym. Unfortunately, I've spoken at the funeral of a young man, in his late twenties, who died as a result of overuse of anabolic agents.

I HOPE YOU always will remember that, no matter what your fitness goals may be, they can be achieved without gimmicks, drugs included. I confess that I am not a very good hand-holder. For the people I train who are not athletes, I feel it is far better to empower them with knowledge and encouragement, and get them to go out on their own. So I hope the following reminders will help you succeed in reaching your fitness goals:

1. Forget the quick fix garbage you see on TV and are emailed or hear about. Becoming fit takes work, but it is work you will enjoy.

2. Your "vision" is based on your desire, and it means everything. When your desire is regularly fed and becomes strong, it causes eating right and training faithfully to dominate laziness and junk food.

3. Don't be afraid to dream big. When you set goals beyond your supposed ability, you'll find the ability you never knew you possessed.

4. Be honest with yourself.

5. Pick things you like to do. It doesn't have to be in the gym. Be creative. This is your journey. Activities such as hiking are available to everyone; even in the city you can find a hundred different routes to take.

6. Set your own goals. They belong to you, and you own them.

7. Make both short-term and long-term goals.

8. Ask for help and encouragement.

9. Incorporate cardiovascular work into your routine.

10. Necessity is the mother of invention, and of success.

Antidote Reminder

Be creative. Activities such as hiking are available to everyone; even in the city, you can find a hundred different routes to take.

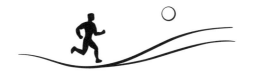

10

Q & A

'Diabetics who are into an exercise routine have to monitor themselves and get an understanding of how to balance insulin against activity . . .'

I CONCLUDE ALL of my speeches and presentations by inviting questions from the audience. Without a doubt this is my favorite part of every appearance; it gives me insight into the audience and gives the audience the chance to ask what they want to know. It's also a great way to make sure I've addressed everything that those in attendance wanted to hear about, and to clear up any confusion my remarks might have caused. Having a Q & A session seems like a good way to wrap up *The Diabetes Antidote,* too. But since a book doesn't afford the opportunity for the spontaneity of crowd participation, I've chosen to present the questions I am asked most often at conferences and clinics, as well as some that have been emailed to me.

How do you exercise if you've had a rough day with blood sugars?

Great question! Life can be complex, and all of you know how difficult it can be if your BG levels have been off. *You* feel poorly and so does your body. The problem is the same for all of us with diabetes, but the key is in your response. First and foremost the answer is that I make the decision that I will go ahead and exercise. When you make this resolve, your follow-through is strengthened; you've decided, period. Most of the time, if things aren't correct, people will wait until their sugar improves. But then something else has come up, and when that happens, it becomes easy just to push it off. It has become instinctive for me: "You know what, I'm going anyway." I correct it on the way to the gym or the track. If it is still off, I'll keep correcting until it's right. We all know the effects a rough day presents, but do you realize how much better you'll feel if you do some type of activity? Incredibly better! Tell yourself, "C'mon, you don't have to do a full workout; just do half of it." Try it! You'll be surprised. I sometimes wind up doing more than I normally would have. So the trick is to take that first step and go. You feel like a conqueror instead of being conquered.

Is there a danger in doing that?

No, because I'm very sure I've got things under control before I start. I've addressed the sugar imbalance, so at that point it's not a question of whether the blood sugar has been addressed. I'm sure I'm safe to proceed and the trick then becomes convincing your "feelings" that you need to go, not complain, even to yourself. Go.

Does it affect your ability to do your workout?

Sure, sometimes it can, but it doesn't always. For the most part, it's not physiological. The effect is because it makes you feel bad. Everyone is different, but with me I usually feel irritated when my sugars are high, and lackluster or a little disoriented if my sugar is low.

Chris Dudley, the pro basketball player, and his wife and I were talking about the misimpression that so many people with diabetes, kids in particular, have. They think,

"You're an athlete. You don't have to struggle with this." I asked Chris, "Do you ever hear this?" Before I had finished my sentence he started shaking his head "yes." We had a long conversation about people who don't understand that just because you succeeded in an athletic endeavor, it doesn't mean you didn't struggle to get there or don't have the same highs, the same lows, the same problems that everybody else has. Chris will tell you this is a vital message to everyone. It makes it so much easier for people to say, "Well if they did it, I can too. They're going through the same crap that I'm going through. They have to correct the lows and, they have to correct the highs."

(By the way, Chris has an excellent basketball camp and foundation. For information about them, go to his Web site, www.chrisdudley.org.)

With the way you train and with your diabetes, are you more prone to highs or lows?

I'm more prone to lows because of my activity level, because I'm burning so many calories. I had quite a bit of difficulty for some time but I've learned to become very careful. My trick is always to try to drop the amount of medication I use – very minutely but consistently. I keep dropping it so that the less body fat I carry, the less medication I need. In this regard the insulin pump is an ideal solution. I'm using insulin to transport the carbohydrates but my body is also running on its own adipose tissue (fat) for fuel, and this is exactly what we want to happen.

I go to the gym with a meter and glucose in my bag. If I'm wearing a pump I'll also drop it in there, too. If I need to correct my sugar levels, it's easy for me because I've

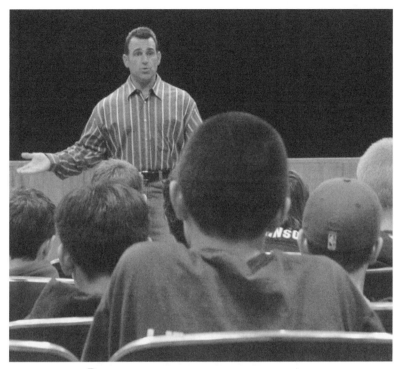

DOUG SPEAKS TO AUDIENCES OF ALL AGES.

brought what I need with me. I'm conscious of all the factors: where my sugars are when I started, how much training I'm doing, how intense and what type of training I'm doing, how long the pump has been off, what I've had prior, and how much insulin I have in my system. It seems complex, but for those of us who compete, it becomes an autopilot response.

Diabetics who are into an exercise routine have to monitor themselves and get an understanding of how to balance their BG levels, the insulin or other medications they use, with the foods they're eating and gauge it against their activity level.

Do you just leave it all to the pump while you're training, just trust the pump to control yourself? Do you have to take it off while you're lifting weights?

Most often, I'll detach the pump when I'm training. Sometimes the motions are too much – if I'm doing cleans and presses with more than 200 pounds, for example. The drop impact can be brutal. (I've already broken one pump doing that.) This is something you will easily get accustomed to. Whether you're working out in a gym or at home, or participating in competitive athletics, it all depends on what kind of activity you're engaged in, and whether or not your pump is going to impede your performance. Either way, you make appropriate adjustments.

Sometimes I'll leave it in and turn it off temporarily if the activity is, say, climbing up a mountainside at a fast pace. When we get up on top, perhaps we want to hike farther. (Last time going through Muir Woods it became a seven-hour trek. I had the pump and some protein bars, and it worked out perfectly). But again, this is a very individualized issue and relies in part on how well you recognize the signs that you're getting low or high.

Are you testing your sugar at the beginning and during your workouts? How do you keep track of how you're doing?

Even though I'm working out so consistently, I still test pretty frequently. The leaner I am, the easier it is to know when a low is coming. I'll feel it. If I've detached the pump and it's 30 minutes into the workout and the low is coming as a result of all the activity I've done, I have to be careful not to overcompensate (too much sugar), because I'll have a smaller amount of insulin later on in my system. I've found it's so much easier in the gym to detach the pump because I make my exercise chase my sugar. For a short time period I rely on my conditioning and the exercise to act as my pump. Let's say I come to the gym and my glucose reading is 89. Not wanting to risk a low with extended cardio, I'll hit the anaerobic training full- bore. (Anaerobic work sometimes elevates blood glucose.) I'll still be careful that I don't drop down, but many times it will become slightly higher, depending on the pace. Afterwards I'll take some whey protein along with a little slow release carbs to begin replenishing my muscle, and jump to the cardio. I push it to keep my metabolism cranked up and the transfer of glucose exercise-induced. An hour or two later, I'm finished. I'll check my sugar, put the pump back on and kick up a bolus to cover the time that I missed. (A bolus is a larger dose of insulin, usually taken before a meal to offset the rise in blood glucose that results from eating.)

Do you let yourself start your workouts with blood glucose that's higher than you would normally maintain?

This depends on the workout. Yes, if it is long-term aerobic work, but not excessively higher. No, if it is anaerobic work. Some people start out in the 200s, but this is mostly event-specific, such as for a marathon. I personally don't like to do this even with cardio, because for me, it creates a poor feeling internally, a kind of nausea. I absolutely do not have elevated sugars if I'm engaging in high intensity training. Besides having that bad feeling inside, it puts a lot of pressure on your vascular system. I prefer to start cardio at 120-170 BG. If it's weights I'm starting with, I prefer to be 80-110. The exact numbers might be 136 or 183 or 92-126.

When you feel a low coming on during a training session, what do you do?

I'll test, and find out how low it is. If it's very low, I'll correct it with a "shot" or sometimes a protein drink with glucose tabs (to help stabilize me long term). A lot of times I'll use Mountain Dew because of its high caffeine. An occasional effect of a low is that the body attempts to save the vital organs and subsequently causes the heart rate to lower and blood pressure to drop. It's doing that to protect the body, but physically, for the activity, it's counterproductive. Caffeine is a stimulant and it indirectly helps advance the uptake of the glucose by sparking the release of adrenalin and thus increasing the heart rate and elevating the blood pressure.

Isn't lifting weights dangerous if you are an older person like me?

Not lifting weights is dangerous for an older person! One of the most dangerous issues older people face is fracturing bones, especially their hips, mostly as a result of falling. This is the primary reason older adults wind up in nursing homes. Women who do not engage in resistance training (such as weight lifting) actually lose bone density. Resistance training coupled with calcium supplements is hands-down the most effective way to offset osteoporosis. The weight training actually enhances the body's uptake of calcium!

To give you an example, after my leg had healed from six fractures I suffered in a freak accident and the surgery I had to undergo to repair them, I gradually but consistently returned to training my legs with heavy work. When the orthopedic surgeon did the second surgery to remove the plate that had been put in my leg, the surgery took an additional two hours of shaving and prying. He said in ten years of surgery I had the hardest bones he has ever worked on. The reason? The heavy training.

Look at Jack Lalane. He's in his 90's and he's still able to do far more pushups than most men half his age! Incredible! Use a variety of activities – running, lifting weights, tennis, stair-climbing. Anything resistance oriented will yield bone-building benefits and stimulate bone formation for you.

If I have diabetes, can I benefit from exercise without losing weight?

Without a doubt. Two people with the same body weight can be two different people altogether. The emphasis is on being active. Activity restores the receptiveness of cell receptors. The cells respond better because the activity forces the body to act in the way it was meant to work. The amount of medication your body needs to function properly will begin to decline.

I've been trying to lose weight for a long time. I go to the gym twice a week and walk some, too, but haven't lost any weight. Is there something wrong with me?

There are two ways I can answer this question. Both begin with, "No, there's nothing wrong with you."

One answer is that you must stop "trying" to lose weight. Instead, make a commitment, and get it done. If you were five-feet-eight and weighed 250 pounds, and I offered you $17,000,000 to lose 100 pounds in eight months, you would find a way. The key is to set your own goals, and make them a reality. You must address the "need" to get the job done, and remind yourself on a daily basis. You can do it.

The second answer is that you need to understand what it takes to lose weight. Don't think you are "exercising" if you are walking around the block with a 650-calorie triple caramel mocha and talking on your cell phone. You must train your body to burn fat. The following simple "Calories In vs. Calories Out" table will get you started:

2,000 calories in – 1,500 calories out = body fat gain
2,000 calories in – 2,000 calories out = no change
2,000 calories in – 2,600 calories out = drop in body fat

Calories out equals the amount of energy you expend with the activity in which you engage, plus the number of calories your body burns while at rest, which is your Basal Metabolic Rate or BMR. Exercise moves your BMR to a higher level than anything else can. Inactivity – and inadequate activity – trains your body to send calories to the fat cells. It slows your metabolism and tells your body you don't need the energy for fuel, so, in effect, "please store it" (as fat). If you had 90 flights of stairs at work, and you had to climb them every day, you'd see a change in the way your body processes food fairly quickly.

How can I lose weight around my stomach?
Let me tell you first what won't work. You can do all the sit-ups you want, or touch your toes as many times as you want, and neither will reduce the size or change the shape of your stomach. It might strengthen your abdominal muscles, depending on how much and how often you do that. But you'll never see those muscles unless you reduce the fat in your stomach area.

The best ways to reduce the fat are by eating a balanced diet, eating in moderation, and engaging in some form of aerobic exercise on a consistent basis. You choose what that aerobic exercise is, but it has to be something you do regularly, and you have to sustain it long enough and at a sufficient intensity that your body is forced to supplement its normal use of insulin by burning some of the fat in your body. Since you're storing a lot of fat cells in your stomach area, you'll start to see it get smaller as you continue your exercise routine along with the changes in your eating habits.

Can your diet work for anyone, or must they be into weightlifting, bodybuilding, or competitive sports?

I understand that you may not want to be "super lean" or super strong. But you do want to lose your fat and strengthen or tone your body to some degree, right? Especially so, if you have diabetes or are trying to avoid developing Type 2, right?

Physique athletes possess the least amount of body fat and some of the most muscular bodies on earth. The principles we use are flawless for losing body fat and gaining muscle. Period. If there was a better way to accomplish this, we and every other athlete would undertake it. Here are the guidelines:

1. Engage in activities that you enjoy; put your focus on doing them regularly.

2. Eat moderate combinations of lean proteins, whole food carbohydrates and good fats (poly and monounsaturated).

3. Eat smaller meals more frequently.

4. Drink far more pure water every day, and you'll see your body fat diminish. Start with a half-gallon minimum. (At 198 to 208 pounds, I use 1.25 to 1.75 gallons a day.)

5. Eat less food and far fewer starchy carbohydrates, especially at nighttime, BUT make the appropriate medication adjustments.

6. Think about your decision and your desires, and commit to eating clean and lean food for your daily life.

7. Allow yourself to eat "fun foods," but make it one or two meals per week.

Antidote Reminder

If your pre-exercise blood glucose isn't perfect, don't get depressed. Fix it on your way to exercise. This follow-through will keep you on the right track.

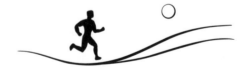

The lessons of April 1, 2007

ON APRIL 1, 2007, I experienced an extreme low blood sugar at a movie theater in Redwood City, CA. As I tried to make it to a concession stand to fix the problem, a security guard thought I was intoxicated and asked me to leave. He called the police when I did not comply. Ultimately I was arrested and charged with assaulting an officer, even though I had lost my vision and had trouble standing.

Perhaps you read or heard about the incident, and are wondering how that could happen to someone who is presenting himself as an authority on exercise, fitness and insulin management. The short answer is that insulin management can be tricky at times for anyone with diabetes, as I have tried to convey in this book and as many with this disease know first hand. There are many lessons to be learned from what happened to me. Briefly, the most important are:

1. A low blood sugar can happen to any diabetic, even if he or she is "under control." In my case, I had switched to a different type of insulin two days prior because my pump, which uses another type of insulin, needed repair. I had exercised that morning, and I misjudged the coupling of the new insulin as well as the amount I needed.

2. There remains a critical need to train and educate our population about the medical complications associated with diabetes, especially the dangers with Type 1. Neither the security guard nor the police officers who responded to this call were familiar enough with the symptoms of low blood sugar. Though I did not smell of alcohol and said I needed sugar, they did not know the difference between the actions of someone who is drunk and a person exhibiting the disoriented, unsteady and unresponsive behavior so common to the low blood sugar condition.

In the controversy my ordeal provoked, I heard from diabetics worldwide who said they have had similar experiences. Their responses argue convincingly for a national campaign to raise awareness and increase understanding regarding diabetes within our society—from law enforcement and public safety to schools and workplaces. I hope my personal encounter helps accomplish that goal. As a first step, Children with Diabetes, the American Diabetes Association and Animas added this incident to their legislative efforts.

To learn about progress on the educational front, I invite you to visit two Internet sites, http://sugarfitness.com and www.thediabetesantidote.com. In the meantime, I have to live what I preach. In this book I tell you to get up and press forward. Just the same, I must step over the embarrassment; correct the injuries instead of bemoan them; and move ahead.

I offer my sincerest thanks to the many people who immediately stood by my side. Jeff, Rick, Richard, Andrea and my brother Brian are tops on that list. Of note, more than a few police officers I know came to my side as well.

D.B.

Co-Author's Note

I AM NOT a diabetic, and I don't want to be one. But I weigh more than I should; I have exercised less than I should for most of my adult life; and there's Type 2 in my family. All of that has made writing *The Diabetes Antidote* with Doug Burns a more beneficial personal experience than I could have imagined when we first discussed collaborating on this book.

Learning about cells and cell receptors, the way insulin works with them to deliver glycogen (and what happens when it doesn't), and how regular activity can improve and sometimes even mimic insulin's efficient performance has changed my appreciation for the value – the importance – of daily exercise.

And hearing Doug's common-sense thoughts on taking personal responsibility for my physical condition has motivated me to an extent I doubted was possible, especially at my age (over 60).

As I worked on this book, I realized that I was writing about myself in many respects. I knew I could be doing more to influence my personal health, and I had to admit there was no excuse for me not to step up. I didn't know as much as I should about how my body works, but once I had a better understanding, what I had to do was obvious.

So, just as Doug recommends, I made a decision; I set a goal; and I committed to following through. I began exercising a minimum of five times a week, starting out at 15 minutes per night on the treadmill and gradually building to 60 minutes within six weeks. I included a modest progression with hand-held weights, started eating the right kind of breakfast, and moderated my lunches and dinners. And I promised myself I would not back off.

I'll never be mistaken for Mr. Universe. But I am confident I have improved my chances of avoiding the onset of Type 2. And that's the point! Anyone can use Doug's antidote to combat diabetes.

I hope his message inspires you as much as it did me.

D.D.

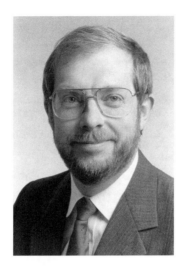

Denny Dressman completed a 43-year career as a newspaper reporter and editor in 2007. Preceding 25 years at the Rocky Mountain News *in Denver, he was an award-winning journalist in Cincinnati, Louisville, and Oakland. He is the author of two previous books,* Gerry Faust: Notre Dame's Man In Motion *(A.S. Barnes, 1980) and* Yes I Can! Yes You Can! Tackle Diabetes and Win! *(ComServ Books, 2005), and has edited and produced several others. He is a past recipient of the Ohio Associated Press Sports Editors' award for Best Sports Column and numerous other writing awards, and is a past president of both the Denver Press Club and the Colorado Press Association. He lives in Denver.*

Acknowledgments

THIS BOOK IS the realization of a different kind of fitness goal, to share with others what I have learned about preventing Type 2 diabetes and limiting the effects of Type 1 through a committed program of regular exercise. I have many people to thank for their support, encouragement, friendship and willingness to share knowledge and expertise. Included are the following members of the medical profession: Dr. Mayer Davidson, whose initial urging opened my mind to the idea of writing a book about exercise for people with diabetes; to Dr. Ed Amento, founder of the Molecular Medicine Research Institute (www.mmrx.org) in Mountain View, CA, for his help and direction; Dr. Andrea Hayes, "The Endo Queen," Type 1 diabetic herself, and invaluable resource for so many patients in Nashville; and Dr. Zhi Yang, for his work with Advanced Glycation End Products.

I also thank Kirk Raab, wise friend, great storyteller, and former CEO of Genentech, creators of Humalin; Vinson Keyhea and "Doc" Rhodes, my original mentors in powerlifting and fitness and close friends still today; Marc Lechner of Nektar Therapeutics; my brother Brian, sister Melissa and Mom and Dad; John Thomas, Ray Campisi, Bill Hooper, Charles Renfroe, Rick Philbin, Bill Davey, Dr. Kevin Jones, Brian Wren, Ricky Greenwald, Kristen Smith, Bob Mallord, Jerry Trout, Diane McQuaid, Martha Metz, Mike Cassidy,

Gerry Shaltz and Dennis Rozniak, for their friendship and help. I would not have made it without them all.

Denny Dressman has his own list. At the top of it, always, is his wife Melanie, a first-rate editor in her own right even though it is not her chosen profession, who read every line of the manuscript at least three times. Her encouragement, belief in the project and constant support are instrumental in its completion. Also, Susan Remkus, for her perceptive and thoughtful attention to the final version of the book; Scott Johnson, whose eye for presentation speaks for itself in this and everything else he touches; and Judy Joseph, founder of Paros Press, whose guiding hand and assistance in so many ways make a book like this one a reality.

Two Important Web Sites

To help people with weight loss and issues related to diabetes management and Type 2 prevention, Doug Burns is launching a new Internet site, **www.sugarfitness.com**, an interpersonal social network dedicated to helping people with diabetes and those trying to lose weight.

Also, anyone interested in fitness-related contests will find **www.fitknox.com** to be the biggest and best international fitness site anywhere.

"Incredibly Inspirational"
— dLife TV

"Highly Recommended"
— children with DIABETES

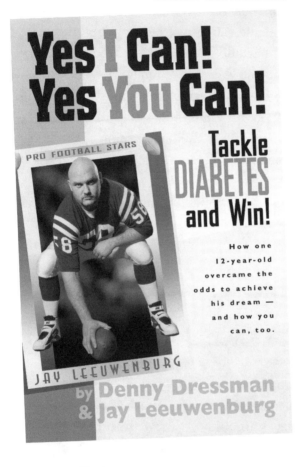

"*As I am getting further into the book, I'm just amazed at the issues and questions it answers, almost like you were reading my mind!*"

"*Thank you so much for this book. It is a God-send.*"

"*I just finished reading your book. It's a keeper!*"

"*I work with newly diagnosed pedi diabetics. I have quotes from the book on my office door that change weekly.*"

Recipient of dLife TV's
Making a Difference in Diabetes Award

Chosen **Best General Health Book** for 2006
by USABookNews.com

"*It's one of the best sports books I've ever read — and certainly the most inspirational.*"
Lance Porter, Editor-in-Chief
Didabetes Postive Magazine

Jay Leeuwenburg was diagnosed with Type I Diabetes only days after his 12th birthday.

From his first day in an unfamiliar Oregon hospital, 2,200 miles from his suburban St. Louis home, Jay's attitude toward living his life to the fullest was, "Yes I Can!"

Blessed with a combination of competitiveness, intelligence, confidence and athletic ability, he took charge of his diabetes, and thus took charge of his life.

Recruited by the University of Colorado after other major colleges were scared away by his diabetes, he started at center on Colorado's national champion team in 1990, then capped his third straight season as a starter by being named first-team center on every All-American team chosen the following year. He played in four bowl games and two national championship games during his career, and was team captain his senior season.

During a 9-year pro career that included 4 seasons with the Chicago Bears, 3 with the Indianapolis Colts and 1 each with the Cincinnati Bengals and Washington Redskins, Jay played with and against Hall of Fame immortals; made headlines as one of pro football's first big-money free agents; and experienced the playoffs as both winner and loser.

"Yes I Can! Yes You Can!" is filled with entertaining and touching stories that will span the range of every reader's emotions. For anyone with diabetes, as well as their family members and friends, it delivers a motivating message that should not be missed.

Yes I Can! Yes You Can!

can be ordered online at
www.yesicanyesyoucan.com
$16.95 + tax and shipping

'An important story'

"This book . . . tells an important story. The word 'inspiring' gets thrown around quite a lot, but I can think of no better word to describe Leeuwenburg's experience with diabetes. His dedication is remarkable, and his accomplishments show it."

– *Writer's Digest*

'Valuable Advice'

"The word 'victim' was never in Jay's vocabulary. Dressman and Leeuwenburg provide encouragement, hope and valuable advice for families dealing with a potentially debilitating disease."

– *The Bonham Group*

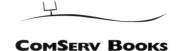

COMSERV BOOKS

To order additional copies of

The Diabetes Antidote

or to learn more about
preventing Type 2 Diabetes
and combatting Type 1

visit our website at
www.thediabetesantidote.com

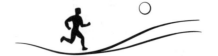